EAT FAT, GET FIT

THE SECRETS TO EATING FAT FOR PERMANENT WEIGHT-LOSS AND PEAK PHYSICAL PERFORMANCE

Author of *Ketogenic Catastrophe*

ERIC STEIN

ACKNOWLEDGEMENTS

First I would like to thank my beautiful wife Holly. Her strength and support has guided me to where I am today, and without her my goals of changing the world would not be possible. Dr. Mark Hyman for writing the incredibly informative *Eat Fat, Get Thin* that inspired this book. Tim Ferriss and Lewis Howes for their amazing podcast's which helped me find my passion in writing. Dave Asprey, Dr. Mark Sircus, Dr. Domonic D'Agostino, and all the other warriors who battle for the health of humanity. Thank you!

Table of Contents

A Fat Introduction

A new paradigm in the health and fitness world has emerged. Weight-loss gurus, fitness junkies, and health experts alike are all saying the same thing: <u>EAT MORE FAT</u>! To most people this sounds crazy. Eating *more fat* couldn't possibly help to lose weight, get fit, or reverse disease. This goes against everything we were told our entire lives. Decades of low-fat health advice has produced a ***fat fear***. The result? We've become scared of steak and butter.

America has taken nutritional advice from prestigious medical associations, governmental agencies, and specialized nutrition experts for half a century, yet we are fatter and sicker than ever. Believe it or not, the average American woman now weighs as much as the average 1960s male! (2) Somewhere along the line we've missed something; a piece to our puzzle. Through no fault of our own, while struggling with the hustle-and-bustle of our daily lives, we bypassed information about proper diet and nutrition. We set our diet on autopilot and walked away from the controls while the skies were clear, never imagining the people we trusted could have been so wrong.

Misleading information has contributed to our subpar dietary framework. The standard nutritionist will tell you *"fat has 9 calories per gram while carbs and protein have only 4, so eat less fat and you will lose weight and feel better."* (1) We've become **calorie crazy**, yet most people don't even know what a calorie is! Ask 100 people and 99 will have no clue. The *Eat Fat, Get Fit* program is here to change that. It will change not only your understanding of calories, but your entire perspective the foods you eat.

This idea that "fat makes you fat" is widely believed to be true. You could say it's matter-of-fact. However, this fact turns to fiction once you understand the basics of human digestion. America has been reducing dietary fat for almost four decades, yet the percentage of people who fat and sick has only increased. It's time we separate fact from fiction. We live in an age of information where anyone can pick up a book like this and learn exciting new ideas. As these ideas spread, we will see the collective health of our people change for the better. Many people, including myself, believe this change is already underway.

Eating more fat is actually one of the best things you can do for yourself, **but there is a method to this madness.** There are rules to follow and ideas to comprehend before simply eating more fat. Before playing

chess you must know how the pieces move, and before eating more fat

you must know how your body will react. *Eat Fat, Get* Fit is here to teach

you the rules of a higher fat lifestyle. It is here to be your guide book;

your yellow brick road to physical health and wellness. It will warn you of

the mistakes made by those who tried and failed before you. Why make

the same mistakes countless people before you have already made? Read

carefully and your reward will be permanent weight-loss, peak physical

fitness, and a life filled with health and vibrancy.

PART I: FAILURE TO FAT

"Looking and feeling sick, tired, fat, or weak is not an

option, and you were not meant to be that way"

-Dave Asprey, Author of The Bulletproof Diet

1. A Short Fat History

Prior to the age of industrialized food very few health experts had a problem with fat. Back when food was food, fat was considered an excellent source of dependable energy. There were no obesity, heart disease, or cancer epidemics. Only humans eating food.

Early in the 1980s, the US Dietary Guidelines warned us about potential dangers of eating too much fat. The guidelines implored the public to reduce their dietary fat intake citing many potential dangers to our health. (1) Around the same time, a connection between dietary fat and excess body fat was made, although this connection was never founded on solid science. We heeded these warnings and began massive reductions in fat, fearing for our lives. The chicken breast with steamed veggies became the iconic weight-loss meal as helpless Americans noticed their midsections starting to expand. The problem was clear; fatty foods were to blame.

In the 1960's 1 out of 100 Americans had type 2 diabetes. Today, that ratio is now 1 in 10; a mind-blowing tenfold increase. In the same timeframe American obesity went from 1 in 7 to 1 in 3, with projections putting that number at 1 in 2 by 2050. (2) Something is terribly wrong. It is interesting that the 60's were also a time of massive expansion in the processed foods market. Long shelf lives became an important part of food production as companies realized that spoiled foods don't sell well. The longer a product could sit on the shelf, the more profitable it was. Shareholders rejoiced as non-perishable foods flooded the market.

As a result, food manufactures came up with new ways of preserving food. The US Dietary Guidelines didn't say much about highly processed or sugar-packed foods, so all avenues were explored to find the best ways to preserve their products. Fat was the boogy man we were warned about, not sugar or processing. Given what we knew at the time, this seemed like a great idea. As my mentor told me; in anything you do, always try to use the least amount of time, energy, resources, and money. That's what these companies started doing.

Their desire for higher profits is not inherently *bad*. Capitalism is in fact one of the reasons America became so great. However, when the public lost interest and turned their attention elsewhere, we missed several warning signs that should have made us rethink the direction our food supply was headed. Currently, the desire for profit has superseded the desire to produce fresh, healthy food. Foods that are high in good fats spoil quickly, and spoiled foods mean spoiled profits. Healthy food has become less profitable, and as we know, America means business. We like to make money, and we are good at it.

Fast forward 30+ years and the wheels of industry have continued to turn. Our stores have become packed with highly processed, high-sugar, low-fat food products that are shelf stable for years. Do we blame capitalism? Nah. Lack of information to the public is to blame. We can go around pointing fingers at medical institutions, government agencies, food producers, and the media all we want, but only when we point the finger back at ourselves do we open the door for change. By pointing the finger at others, we give them power over us.

Eat Fat, Get Fit will help you take this power back where it belongs, in your hands. We live in an age of information where anyone can pick up a book like this and learn about their health. What you get from this book is not weight-loss, but power. <u>Information is power</u>. Information will allow you to make the choices you didn't know you had, and these choices will ultimately lead to your weight-loss and physical fitness goals.

Our history has already been written; there's no changing it now. Our goal must be to understand the mistakes of our past in order to make the right decisions for our future. We must understand our *fear of fat* so that we can overcome it. As we continue down this rabbit hole I urge you to keep an open mind, but also maintain a healthy sense skepticism. Remember, our lack of skepticism is what got us here in the first place...

KEY POINTS

- ➢ **Before industrialized food, fat was a normal part of our diets**
- ➢ **Diabetes has increased TENFOLD while we reduced fat intake**
- ➢ **Obesity now reaches 1-in-3 Americans**
  - ○ **Projected to be 1-in-2 by 2050**
- ➢ **Shelf-stable, high-carb foods are more profitable**
- ➢ **We possess the power to make the changes necessary in our lives**

2. Fear Behind the Fat

If someone asked you what foods you were *afraid* of, what would you say? Cheeseburgers? Pastries? Brussels sprouts? It's not often we talk about fear and food at the same time, but to fully embrace the principles of *Eat Fat, Get Fit*, we must be willing to acknowledge an underlying fear that many of us have naturally developed. For decades we've been told fat will harm us, make us obese, and steal our vitality. Doctors have been recommending low-fat diets to promote weight-loss and a healthy life, and the media seems to run constant headlines connecting fat to heart attacks and strokes. A fear has been created deep down in our minds.

This fear of fat has become deeply engrained in our culture as well, all the way down to the words we use. Have you ever considered the multiple meanings of the word "FAT" and the feelings it produces? For example, we label people fat if they are overweight. In this instance, the word fat is being used as a description of our *physical nature*. This physically descriptive use of the word fat produces a subconscious emotional fear which can manifest in dietary choices. This fear is incredibly dangerous to those who wish to lose weight.

When we decide it's time to lose weight, we are faced with the option of eating protein, carbohydrates, and....**FAT**. This is where the emotional fear can manifest. Regardless of what you read in some diet book, if you think you are *fat*, are you are less likely to eat more fat. Period. This has nothing to do with the physical effects of fat on your body, but plays directly to your emotional side. Fat is bad. Fat on your body is bad, so fat in your food is bad. In what universe have you ever heard a nutritionist say fat is good? Unfortunately, for millions who struggle with excess body fat, this **emotional fear** may stop weight-loss in its tracks.

As a response to this fear, dietary fat has been labeled a *public enemy* by government organizations, and a war against it has ensued, thus reinforcing the fat-fear. Much like the war on drugs, poverty, and terrorism has only increased these problems, the war on American obesity seems to have produced more obesity. The statistics don't lie. The Center for Disease Control (CDC) has projected U.S. adult obesity to hit 1 in 2 by 2030. (1) Terrorism has spread across the globe, poverty and drug abuse continue to skyrocket, and the American population has gotten fatter by the year. There is a pattern here for those who wish to see it.

This is not to say a lack of fat is the *cause* of heart disease, only that statistics have shown decreasing fat intake has not stopped it. We've been told saturated fat intake is associated with cardiovascular disease, yet recent studies have shown the opposite. As we continue to eat loads of processed foods and refined carbohydrates, sugar being the biggest culprit, heart disease will remain amongst the biggest threats to the developed world. (2-4)

CAN SCIENCE SQUASH THE FEAR?

Many are beginning to realize turning to "science" for definitive answers on diet and nutrition has become somewhat difficult. The National Institute of Health has a database chocked full of conflicting research papers which confuse rather than clarify anything about diet. It is a melting pot of truth and half-truths, and almost impossible tell the difference between the two. Twenty studies will say fat is bad while twenty others will say it's good. The outcomes seem to be determined by who funded them, which has shaken our trust in science.

This doesn't mean science is *bad*, or that it can't ever be trusted, only that it has been *compromised,* and we must look in multiple areas to find the truth that works for us. The scientific process is beautiful, but political, economic, and financial interests do not sit idly by while science runs its course. Money and power can easily upset the delicate process of true science. Even if there were no manipulation or corruption, people get things wrong. It happens all the time. In fact, it has happened all throughout history. Do you recall doctors recommending their favorite brand of cigarettes?

So where are we supposed look if science can't give us definitive answers? The writing on the wall is clear; we must learn to look **inward** for the answers we seek. We must be willing to test hypotheses ourselves and determine if something is true or false. For example, I read the hypothesis that fat is good for you and will help with losing weight, so I decided to test this hypothesis on myself. What followed was the most dramatic weight-loss of my life, and in record time! My wife and I shed 30 pounds each within five months. This was the result of looking inward for answers.

It seems like a paradox, but as I get older I have become stronger and more resilient. I have realized a level of physical performance I thought would only be available as a teenager. This has occurred as I've

decreased the amount of exercise I do. The key variable has been my adaptation of a higher fat diet; and I am not alone.

The first step in making this transition is to let go of your *"fat fear."* In order to realize the benefits a high-fat diet has to offer, you must acknowledge your unwarranted fear of fat. As silly as it may sound, acknowledging your fear is what ultimately leads to overcoming it. In the next chapter we will confront the second major hurdle to overcome in your *Eat Fat, Get Fit* journey; your sweet tooth. The *fat fear* is priority #1, but your *sweet tooth* is undoubtedly #2.

KEY POINTS

> - We have developed a "FAT FEAR"
> - Heart disease, diabetes, and cancer have <u>increased</u> as we <u>decreased</u> fat intake
> - The word <u>fat</u> carries unconscious emotional baggage
> - "Science" is currently not a reliable source of dietary advice
>   - Who funded the research often determines the results
>   - Testing on yourself is the only way to know what is right FOR YOU

3. Sweet Misery

Imagine standing in line at the grocery store, minding your own business, when suddenly there's a tap on your shoulder. You spin around, confused as to why someone would bother you, but no one is there. Instead of a nosey stranger, a giant rack of candy sits there silently, almost *begging* you to investigate its bounty of chocolaty goodness.

"Don't do it" you think immediately.

"You don't need that candy bar….it's BAD for you."

"…but oh wow…10 for $10! That's a great deal!"

Gotcha. The imaginary tap on your shoulder turned into three candy bars, one of which is getting eaten on the way home for sure. Before you know it, 30 to 40 grams of sugar surges through your veins. You feel fantastic. Energy levels are up, motivation is up, and you can feel that pep back in your step. After a long day at work you deserved that *reward*.

The title of this chapter may sound a bit embellished, but its content aims to paint a detailed picture of the biggest struggle many people face. Everyone knows deep down that candy bars are not going to help you lose weight, yet we often still indulge ourselves. Why?

Unbeknown to most, sugar activates reward mechanisms in the body that

are both physical and emotional, and unless you pay close attention, they

can easily sabotage weight-loss efforts. Missing these cues from your

body will leave you vulnerable to the automatic reactions that occur

because of this reward system. These emotional decisions can easily run

the majority of your life, and as we'll find out shortly, this is bad news for

weight-loss.

The emotional stress from a long day at work disappears the

instant that candy bar hits your mouth. Gone is the thought of your boss

yelling at you an hour ago about something you forgot to do. Screw him

anyways, he's always yelling about something.   Any anxiety or

uncertainty in your life vanishes instantly as that delicious piece of

chocolaty heaven hits your taste buds. All is right in the world. This is

your *emotional* reward, and it is unrivaled in its power. Even if you are

preoccupied in traffic, talking to your kids or spouse, or working on a

project, and don't actually take the time to enjoy the candy bar, this

emotional reward is still occurring in the background. It always happens.

The physical reward gets your ass back in gear after a tiresome day on the job. Imagine you just worked nine hours and haven't eaten since lunch, and it was a small wimpy lunch that you were less than excited about. Low energy levels mean low blood sugar. As that first heavenly bite of candy bar hits your lips, signals are sent to the brain letting it know an enormous amount of sugar, or glucose, is on the way. There is no longer a need to conserve energy and **feel tired** because blood sugar is about to rise, dramatically. It is quite amazing to sit back and analyze the process as it happens. The body uses these signals, or feedback loops, to keep our systems running as efficiently as possible.

Mother Nature has been refining our bodies for millions of years, but only recently, with the advent of refined sugar, have we been able to spike blood sugar levels so high, and so often. These massive blood sugar spikes, followed by the subsequent plunges, have created a monster that many deem to be the western world's greatest threat. That may sound over-the-top or hysterical, but when you look at the bigger picture, the biggest killer of western citizens are obesity related diseases, all of which are negatively impacted by refined sugars. The title *Sweet Sweet Misery* doesn't sound overly dramatic when looked at from this context.

THE JUNK FOOD JUNKIE

Junkies come in all shapes and sizes. The shopping junkie, the coffee junkie, and the methamphetamine junkie to name a few. The last time I stopped drinking coffee it felt like a semi-truck hit me. I had a pounding headache, was beyond fatigued, and my crankiness levels were through the roof. My wife demanded she be out of town the next time I try to give it up. There is no doubt I am a coffee junkie.

Comparing candy bars to narcotics sounds a bit ridiculous. *"A crack pipe is not as bad as a candy bar"* says my Mom. Bless her soul. However, it is important we address some similarities between the two before moving forward. The goal here is not to *scare* you, but rather create awareness around a <u>negative feedback loop</u> that may be operating in your life. You must first be aware of the problem before you can solve anything.

After consuming a mega-dose of sugar from something like a soda or candy bar, your brain releases a blast of **dopamine** from an area called the Nucleus Accumbens, (1) which is the body's "reward system." It is interesting to note that cocaine and heroin also trigger massive releases of dopamine in this area of the brain. In fact, one of the major components of ANY addiction (drugs, sex, shopping, etc) is the body's desire for this large-scale dopamine release.

What happens when we don't get these precious dopamine hits? Crankiness, headache, body ache, restlessness, fatigue, depression, even night-sweats and anxiety. (2) The level or strength of these symptoms can vary for each person, but they will generally correlate with how much dopamine was being produced and for how long. The person who drinks 64oz of soda per day may have more severe symptoms than one who drinks only 12oz. This is similar to the pack-a-day smoker having a harder time quitting than the pack-a-week smoker. The same principle is in effect. However, everyone's brain chemistry is different, so it's impossible to tell if this will be a problem for you.

The best course of action, as with any addiction, is to taper off slowly. If you consume 100+ grams of refined sugars per day, dropping this down to only 10 or 20 may trigger withdrawal symptoms. While generally not as powerful as heroin, these symptoms should not be taken lightly. A slow decrease in your refined sugar intake over the course of 2-3 weeks is ideal. When you feel like you've gotten to a point of clarity, eliminate refined sugars completely and watch your life change in ways you never imagined. A new world of health, happiness, mental clarity, and vibrancy awaits you on the other side of refined sugar.

Our struggle with sugar is real. Simply look at the obesity and chronic disease epidemics that have gripped the western world. The white powdery substance that kills most people on this planet is not cocaine or heroin, but <u>refined sugar</u>. While its toxicity doesn't match that of heroin or cocaine, its social acceptance and sheer volume of use is what makes it so dangerous.

It is important to understand you cannot *Eat Fat, Get Fit* **while consuming tsunami levels of sugar. It simply will not work. You will likely GAIN weight if fat intake is increased without a reduction in refined sugars.** This addictive aspect of sugar MUST be tackled as you progress with the *Eat Fat, Get Fit* program. If you find yourself having trouble laying off the sugar, take out a pen and paper and quickly write down some reasons you wish to give it up. Read these out loud. Encourage yourself. Ask for help if you need it. Dropping sugar may seem tough, but I promise you it gets easier as time goes on. If you feel a lapse in willpower, go look yourself in the mirror and tell yourself of how strong you are. Motivate yourself. Believe in yourself. Before you know it you will break free from this sweet, sweet misery. Next up, let's take a look at how sugar makes you fat.

SUGAR - INSULIN - BODY FAT

The average 12oz soda contains 39grams of sugar, an almost unbelievable 9 teaspoons, and many people consume 2-3 of these a day! Imagine eating 27 teaspoons of sugar! After consuming a massive amount of sugar, particularly in liquid form, a massive **insulin** response must follow in order to bring blood sugar back down. And guess what? INSULIN SENDS SIGNALS TO THE BODY TO STORE FAT. (3) Go ahead and raise your hand if you are reading this book because you want to store more fat. Anyone? I didn't think so. Not only does it put your body in fat STORAGE mode, but the sheer size of the insulin response creates an extreme stress on the pancreas. This sugar-insulin-body fat feedback loop is important to understand.

AWARENESS EXERCISE

My wife and I often talk about the difference between "thinking you know" and "knowing you know." Sometimes, in order to really believe something, you have to see it right in front of you. This is where the old saying *seeing is believing* comes from. If you see yourself as a visual/hands-on type person and consume large amounts of sugar, do the following awareness exercise. This will burn the image into your mind and help you make better decisions in the future.

Go find your favorite sugary snack or drink and determine how much sugar it contains. If you enjoy a 32oz soda, you'll be looking at around 104 grams of sugar, or about 24 teaspoons. A candy bar can have around 40g of sugar, or about nine teaspoons. After you figure it out, take this same amount of sugar and put it on a plate in front of you.

Now, as you stare at the Mount Everest sized pile of sugar, imagine eating it. **All of it**. Teaspoon by teaspoon. No water to dilute it, no chocolate to put it in. Teaspoon by teaspoon you'll have to eat the entire plate. Can you imagine putting 9 teaspoons of sugar in your mouth and trying to swallow?

What would happen if you tried to do it? Extreme stomach pain and vomiting would likely occur before getting through one soda's worth of sugar. Imagine the trick we are playing on our bodies as we gulp down those sweet, bubbly "soft" drinks. There doesn't seem to be anything "soft" about them.

The good news is you have a choice. You are more powerful than you give yourself credit. You have the ability to change your life at any moment. This change in lifestyle doesn't happen overnight and requires work and dedication. As we know, *nothing worth having is easy*. It requires forgiving yourself when you screw up and drink a soda or eat a candy bar. In fact, it DEMANDS that you cut yourself some slack and allow the process to happen. Be kind to yourself, ask for help if you need it, and remind yourself of why you wish to create change in the first place. **Your success is determined by your ability to overcome failure**.

KEY POINTS

- Sugar addiction is real
  - The body undergoes similar patterns as cocaine and heroin addiction
  - There are physical AND emotional withdrawal symptoms
  - These can easily lead to relapse and failure to lose weight
- Modern diets have dramatically increased sugar intake
- One soda has 9 TEASPOONS of sugar

- o This is almost impossible to eat by itself in one sitting
- ➤ Tapering off sugar is the best way to quit
  - o Cold-turkey can lead to withdrawal symptoms
  - o 2-3 weeks is ideal for tapering
- ➤ Becoming <u>aware</u> is the first step towards beating sugar
- ➤ YOU CAN DO THIS!!

PART II: LET'S GET THE

FATS STRAIGHT

"The **doctor** of the future will no longer treat the human frame with drugs, but rather will **cure** and prevent disease with **nutrition**.

-Thomas Edison

4. Good Fat, Bad Fat?

What comes to mind when you hear the phrase "good-fat?" Do visions of avocado slices appear in your mind? How about olive oil or almonds? This good fat vs. bad fat debate has been raging for years with no end in sight. Wild claims like "heart healthy" have been assigned to fats that are nothing of the sort, as in the case of modern vegetable oils. The purpose of *Eat Fat, Get Fit* is to present a different perspective, or definition, of the word "good" so that you may apply it to your daily life.

There are several factors to consider when determining if a fat source is "good" or not, and these factors differ depending on where the fat comes from (ex. oils, nuts, dairy, meat, etc). There are different levels of quality too. Imagine a 1-10 scale, with 10 best the best version. Two versions of the same fat can show up on different levels of the scale. For example, a cheap version of almond butter can be a 7, while another, higher quality version, shows up as a 10. Under the lid they are both almond butter, but one of them contains more beneficial nutrients and fewer additives, thus giving it the higher score. Generally speaking, the "closer to natural" a fat is, the higher on the scale it will be. Highly processed fats usually show up in a 5 or below, while naturally occurring fats are in the 8-10 range.

The aim here is to give you a basic conceptual understanding of what these factors mean and why they matter. Once you understand the logic behind your choice, you will have an easier time making the right one. Now, let's analyze three different foods that are excellent sources of fat. These foods will have the same name, but as you will see, <u>how they are made</u> will change their score.

To start, let's consider the difference between two versions of butter. Butter is a wonderful source of fat that provides numerous nutritional benefits. In fact, coffee blended with butter is how I start almost every morning. However, when removed far enough from its natural state, it becomes something to be avoided.

> **Grass-fed / pasture-raised butter** - Cows are meant to eat grass, not corn, soy, animal byproducts, or anything else. They are meant to graze in a field with access to fresh air and space to roam. The butter from a cow fed grass is high in vital nutrients that promote health and fitness. [1,2,3]

> **Commercial butter** - 90+% of the butter found in the store is commercial grade. These cows are raised in confined areas, often never seeing the light of day. They are fed grains (which their

digestive systems are not designed for) and are regularly given antibiotics and hormones which end up in the butter. They become sick and deficient in nutrients, thus producing nutrient deficient butter. (4)

The first version of butter comes from a cow that ate its natural diet of grass. This may not seem extraordinary, but studies have shown it is higher in vital nutrients like CLA, butyrate, and various omega-3 fatty acids, which will assist in weight-loss. Also, if the cow has outdoor access it receives numerous benefits from sunlight and exercise. Cows benefit from sunlight just like humans do. The other butter generally comes from a cow that was confined its whole life, fed genetically engineered corn and soy, and often lived in its own waste. It will be less nutritious and less beneficial to your weight-loss and fitness goals.

In our next example, let's look at an excellent snack food many of us often abuse; nuts and seeds. These can be a wonderful tool when trying to slim down and shape up, but it is important to target the best options in order to receive maximum benefits. Consider the difference between the follow options:

Raw or sprouted nuts/seeds - These nuts are not heated above 118° which keeps more of their nutrients intact. They are an excellent source of fat and protein. Many are jam-packed with the super-mineral magnesium and contain plant sterols that may help lower bad cholesterol. Add sea salt to these and you have a powerful and nutrient dense snack. (5)

Canned roasted nuts/seeds - These are by far the most widely available and commonly consumed. What most people don't see is that these nuts and seeds can be covered in vegetable oil and refined salt, and are commonly FRIED not roasted. This allows producers to use old nuts while also ensuring they taste great so you won't stop eating them, quickly needing to buy more. (6)

These seemingly similar foods can have very different outcomes on your body. One version will work towards your weight-loss goals and the other will move you away from them.

Olive oil is the final example we will look at. These two common options are found almost anywhere, and will be sitting right next to each other on the store's shelf. They will likely have similar packaging, and may even come from the same company! To spot the difference, you need to pay attention to the following key words:

Organic, cold-pressed - Organic means no chemicals were used in growing the olives, and cold-pressed means the olives were *pressed* at low temperatures in order to extract the oil. It is more time consuming to press the olives and thus more expensive, but this process leaves more of the nutrients intact,(7) and will pay dividends to your weight-loss efforts.

Non-organic, refined - These olives may have been sprayed with pesticides and insecticides which can end up in the oil. The extraction method is much faster and more efficient, but also involves high-heat, which damages some beneficial nutrients in the oil. Some oil extraction methods utilize harmful chemicals in the process which may be ending up in the oil. (8) While this olive oil is an excellent source of fat, your system may have to overcome these other contaminants as well, thus slowing weight-loss.

Are you beginning to see the bigger picture of how one version of a food can be beneficial while another may actually be doing your body harm? Notice how in each of these comparisons, one option is further from its "natural" state than the other. Generally speaking, the more processing that occurs during production, the further away from natural it becomes, and the less nutritional value the fat will retain. One of the foundational principles of *Eat Fat, Get Fit* is to always choose the best source of fat when possible. Not all fat is created equal, and if we wish to cultivate maximum weight-loss, we must learn to target the best options of fat available. Now, let's take a quick look at what fats to avoid.

THE BAD

Don't think of bad as "evil." Vegetable oils like soybean, corn, canola, cottonseed, safflower, and grapeseed are not the devil, but they should be avoided when possible. These mass-produced oils are higher in omega-6 fatty acids and lower in heart-healthy omega-3's. Due to the processing methods used, many of them contain harmful byproducts of production.

Mass produced canola oil is a perfect example of how wrong things can go. This mass production brings cost down but also opens the door to dramatic drops in quality. High heat and various industrial chemicals, such as cancer causing hexane, can be used in its production.

Many health experts believe that these oils are not fit for human consumption. Even if you find cold-pressed (thus lower yield and more expensive) versions of canola oil, there still remains the issue of excess omega-6 fatty acids. It is best to avoid canola.

Many of these oils have been incorrectly labeled as "heart-healthy" by modern medicine and the media. A common claim is that these vegetable oils contain less saturated fat, so they must be better for your heart. Oxidation, chemical contamination, and genetically engineered ingredients are ignored, along with their lack of heart healthy omega-3s. New data being made available has linked overconsumption of these low quality oils to serious ailments including heart disease and cancer. (9)

THE GOOD

So what exactly is good fat? Everyone may have their own opinion, but the *Eat Fat, Get Fit* follows the paradigm that closest to natural is the best option. Naturally occurring fat is a 10 on the scale.

Avocados are a powerful tool for weight-loss. They are a superfood packed with vitamins and minerals while also containing a hefty serving of fat! They are a fruit with fat! Many claim avocado to be nature's perfect food. Add these to smoothies, salads, breakfast, lunch, and dinner. Everywhere you can.

Cold-pressed, virgin oils like **coconut** and **olive oil** are also extremely beneficial. Use coconut oil in smoothies, for sautéing veggies, or cooking eggs. Olive oil is great as a salad dressing or the base of a sauce.

Grass-fed butter can be used for just about everything. It is great for cooking eggs, adding to potatoes or rice, and even a perfect addition to a smoothie. My personal favorite method for using grass-fed butter is to blend it with coffee as a creamer alternative. Grass-fed butter is exceptionally high in conjugated linoleic acid (CLA) and butyrate. CLA may actually help lower body fat percentages in humans and even fight cancer! Butyrate can fight inflammation, improve gut health, and was shown to make rats resistant to becoming obese! (10-14) From personal experience I can tell you my body fat percentage dropped dramatically when my butter intake increased.

Ghee (clarified butter) is an excellent alternative for those with dairy sensitivities. It has a higher smoke point than butter which makes it safer for higher temperature cooking.

Animal Lard has been used for millennia by humans. Use lard for frying potatoes or cooking veggies; pretty much anywhere you would use oil. Sourcing lard is similar to sourcing animal meat or dairy. The animals given the best conditions to live and food to eat will produce the best lard. Commercial grade lard may contain harmful contaminants and be deficient in nutrients. Remember to consider the source when purchasing, or simply make your own using a slow cooker.

Raw or Sprouted nuts and seeds are also fantastic sources of fat. Most nuts have been pasteurized, roasted, or fried, all of which use high temperatures. Raw versions will contain more nutritional value. Nut-butters like almond and cashew butter make for a delicious snack when paired with your favorite veggies. Peanut butter is up for debate as it contains more omega-6 fatty acids, pose allergy risks, and have been shown to contain higher mycotoxin levels than other nuts. But if you simply can't do almond butter, an organic sugar-free peanut butter will work.

So what is "good fat?" Basically, it comes from the *oldest version* of the food we know. Modern production has been used to dramatically increase output, maximize profits, and extend shelf lives, but this has come at the **expense** of nutritional value. Often times these "new and improved" processes add harmful contaminants which ultimately cause your body to GAIN weight instead of shedding it. *Eat Fat, Get Fit* is concerned with <u>increasing</u> the good fat while <u>decreasing</u> the bad fat. Combine that principle with limited sugar consumption and you have yourself a POWERFULL combination for physical transformation.

KEY POINTS

- ➤ "Good Fat"
    - ○ The closer to natural the better
    - ○ The higher the *quality*, the better the fat
    - ○ Fats higher in omega-3 fatty acids are better
    - ○ Pasteurization can harm the fat
- ➤ "Bad Fat"
    - ○ High in omega-6 and low in omega-3 fatty acids
    - ○ Commercial/industrial production
    - ○ Chemical contaminants
- ➤ The SOURCE of the fat often determines its quality
    - ○ Example:
        - ▪ Grass-fed butter = Good
        - ▪ Grain-fed butter = Bad

5. Meat, Dairy, and Eggs

The *Eat Fat, Get Fit* program harnesses the power of compounding. In other words, repeated action over time will increase your results exponentially. The professional baseball player is good at the game because of the compounding effects of his practice. The phrase "practice makes perfect" comes from this idea. This concept of compounding transfers directly into your dietary choices as well. Practice with diet leads to the perfect body you desire. As we discuss meat, dairy, and eggs, the reader must consider both positive and negative compounding effects if they are to get the entire picture of *Eat Fat, Get Fit*.

Consider the difference between the pack-a-day smoker and the pack-a-week smoker. In whose shoes would you rather be at the end of five years? The reason you would rather be the pack-a-week smoker is because you understand the concept of negative compounding effects. Smoking is bad, so the less you smoke, the better off you are. It's simple. On the flip side, in whose shoes would you rather be at the end of five years; the person who ate healthy food once-a-day for five years or once-a-week for five years? The once-a-day person of course. Again, another simple answer. This means you also understand the concept of positive compounding effects. Keeping this in mind, let's take a look at our meat, dairy, and eggs.

A MEATY MESS

There are indeed dangers of consuming modern day meat, but not for the reasons you think. Fat cells store toxins. (1) It is a protection mechanism to keep harmful contaminants away from vital organs (brain, heart, lungs, etc). If an animal, let's say a cow, lives in a highly toxic environment and eats highly toxic food, this animal's fat will contain higher levels of toxins. There is a real difference between the ribeye steak from a cow raised in a factory-farm versus one raised comfortably outdoors and allowed to eat its natural diet of grass. Many health experts consider these to be two different foods altogether. (2)

The key to getting good fat from your meat is selecting the right meat in the first place. Factory-farmed meat is often tainted with antibiotics and hormones and is higher risk for bacterial contamination. When animals are forced to live in confined areas and not given the space they need to live, the result is low quality meat. This meat is lower in vitamins and minerals and higher in toxic contaminants. (3) The lower quality meat is cheaper to buy because it's cheaper to make. However, you will pay for it in the long run in the form of increased health care costs and sick days from work. This is the result of negative compounding.

The cow allowed to live outdoors, eat a natural diet of grass, and soak in the sun's beneficial rays, will produce meat that is low in contaminants and high in <u>vitamins and minerals</u>. The fat found on this meat is an excellent source of heart healthy, weight-loss promoting omega-3 fatty acids. Many stores carry these grass-fed options, and if your local store does not, you can now easily order it online and have it shipped to your house via companies like US Wellness Meats. The positive compounding effects of consuming this higher quality meat pay huge dividends to your weight-loss efforts.

Modern chicken has taken a turn for the worse as well. Consumer Reports recently ran a story on chicken farming exposing how many major operations were feeding **arsenic** to the chickens in an attempt to fatten them up. If you recall, toxins, such as arsenic, are stored in **fat**. While the amount that eventually ends up on your plate may be small, this does not make eating things like arsenic safe. Why? Because of the power of negative compounding over time. Consuming small amounts of toxins over a long period of time will surely take its toll on your health.

The best form of chicken is labeled pasture-raised and organic. As with cows, outdoor access and a healthy diet will produce meat high in essential nutrients, and the organic label means there will be fewer toxins present. The chicken stuffed in a warehouse next to 10,000 of his friends, never seeing the light of day, and being fed toxins, will not produce healthy meat. Remember, with *Eat Fat, Get Fit*, we are always aiming for the best versions of food whenever possible. These principles hold true for all poultry.

Fish is often glossed over when discussing meat, probably because most people think all fish is the same. Farm-raised fish have begun to fill our meat departments because they are cheaper, easier to get, and come with a nice profit margin (sound familiar?). However, raising fish in confined areas and feeding them things like corn and soy is devastating to their systems. As with the other meats above, taking fish from their natural habitat and diet has made them deficient in vital nutrients. It has also resulted in outbreaks of strange viruses, as was the case recently with farm-raised salmon in Chile. (4) Farmed salmon must be dyed orange or pink because the meat no longer carries its trademark color that results from eating crustaceans such as shrimp and krill. Instead, colorants like canthaxanthin and astaxanthin are added to their feed (imagine a bag of pellets dumped into a pond) in an attempt to mimic this color. (5) Most people never think to look, but next time you find yourself in the grocery store, take a moment to study the difference between farm-raised and wild caught salmon. You will be able to see the difference with your eyes.

The *Eat Fat, Get Fit* program considers the source of meat and fat to be of utmost importance. Meat is an excellent source of fat and protein for the body. It contains many vitamins and minerals as well as being one of the few foods that contains <u>complete proteins.</u> The better your meat is treated, the better it will treat you.

DAIRY DO's AND DON'T's

Dairy has been debated back and forth for years. First it's good, then bad, then low-fat was ok, now grass-fed is best. Even the raw-dairy movement has recently made a resurgence with multiple products available in many grocery stores. It's safe to say that there is no consensus on dairy. So what does that mean for you?

There are a few things we know for sure about dairy. For starters, high-quality dairy will have a greater nutritional value than low-quality dairy. This is actually a theme with all food; the closer to natural the better. The milk that underwent **less processing** is better than the milk that is *highly processed* (pasteurized, homogenized, preserved with sugar, cows fed grains, etc). Cows that eat a natural cow diet (grass) produce higher quality milk than the cows fed genetically engineered corn, soy, and other *miscellaneous* ingredients. This is why grass-fed butter has taken the health communities by storm.

Secondly, we also know a percentage of people will still respond poorly to dairy even when consuming the highest quality versions. Genetic factors could be at play here; or perhaps even some unknown environmental or emotional issues. Whatever the reason, you may be a person who doesn't respond well to dairy. There are two ways to determine if you are one of these people:

1. Give up dairy for 30 days and to see if you feel better. This is the hardest but also most rewarding option because you will feel a sense of accomplishment, even if you don't feel better from

eliminating milk. And of course you could feel both accomplished AND better; an epic double-whammy.

2. Go to your doctor and get a dairy allergy test. This may or may not be conclusive.

While writing this book I completed a 30-day no dairy challenge. My objective was to see if I could notice any positive benefits in how I feel when I didn't consume any. I failed several times in the beginning and had to restart the challenge. In the end it took 38 days to complete, and I didn't see or feel any changes. Now I'm back on the dairy train. Giving up dairy for 30 days may sound hard, and it is, for the first week. After you find your groove using a butter substitute like ghee, it becomes much easier, and actually kind of fun.

Raw, grass-fed, full-fat dairy is the best option if you are going to consume it. If you can't find the raw version, then grass-fed and organic is most preferable. Always choose the whole option of milk. Skim milk is missing the good fat that will help with your weight-loss efforts.

EGG-CELLENT

My wife loves eggs. Scrambled, over easy, over medium, hard boiled, deviled, she loves them all. And I'm glad she loves them, because she's pregnant right now and eggs are amongst the most nutritionally dense foods on the planet. Particularly the yolks. (6) They are a treasure trove of vitamins, minerals, and fatty acids. Eggs are also one of the few foods that contain vitamin D naturally. This makes most people... *eggstatic.* Ok no more egg puns, I'm sorry.

The idea that cholesterol causes heart disease seems to be the biggest fear surrounding eggs. Dr. Dwight Lundell, one of the world's most renowned heart surgeons, in his book *The Cure for Heart Disease: Truth Will Save a Nation,* has a very different opinion about this. He points the finger at inflammation, not cholesterol, as the culprit. (7) There are 20 other books written by 20 other doctors along with a wealth of supporting research to make any sane person doubt the cholesterol-heart disease connection. Cholesterol is actually one of the building blocks of life. It is an energy carrier, and we've been consuming it for millennia. With statin medications being one of the top prescriptions in this country, it's no wonder egg consumption is down.

Similar to meat and dairy, eggs have their best version you should target. Like the others, the closer to Mother Nature the better. If your egg comes from a chicken that lives in a dark warehouse crammed next to

10,000 other chickens, living in their own waste, being fed chemical laden feed, and force fed antibiotics and/or growth hormones, you are going to have what's called a "dead-egg." Dead eggs are lacking in vitamins and minerals as can be seen by their brittle shells due to a lack of calcium. (8) They often crack in the carton or crumble in your hand when hit on the side of a pan. The cost to produce dead eggs is much lower, which is very enticing to profit driven food producers and cost conscious consumers.

High quality eggs come from chickens with access to outdoors, are allowed to peck bugs and critters found on the ground, and are not forced to live in the waste of thousands of other chickens. These are generally labeled "pasture-raised." Their shells are much harder to crack because they are higher in calcium, and the yolks have a dark orange color as opposed to a bright yellow. Don't be fooled by catchphrases like "cage-free" and "vegetarian fed" as these are largely meaningless. Cage-free is mostly just a marketing gimmick, and chickens in nature are NOT VEGETARIANS. They actually thrive on bugs and small insects, and taking these away from them is detrimental to their health.

The cost for pasture-raised eggs is going to be higher, but this is only because demand has not grown enough. As demand for high quality eggs increase, supply will follow and prices will come down, and this is already happening. The Ralph's next to my house now carries two options of pasture-raised eggs. We must remember to allocate our resources (money) properly, and if that means cutting back on other expenses to ensure we have high quality food, then this step <u>must</u> be taken. Making excuses about cost will get us nowhere.

As you move forward with *Eat Fat, Get Fit*, keep in mind the idea of compounding. Eating one carton of pasture-raised eggs, or one pound of grass-fed beef will not make excess weight fly off overnight. True weight-loss and wellness is achieved over time, and compounding is the mechanism by which you achieve it. It may take a bit longer, but these results will be permanent, as opposed to get-fit-quick schemes that often end up leaving you worse off than when you started. Permanent weight-loss is a marathon, not a sprint.

KEY POINTS

- ➢ **Modern commercial farming has made most meat, dairy and eggs deficient in vital nutrients**
- ➢ **Grass-fed, pasture-raised, and organic meat is best**
  - ○ **Cows (all animals actually) fed their natural diet are higher in nutrients**

- ➢ Raw, grass-fed, organic, dairy is optimal
  - ○ Grass-fed organic is next best
  - ○ Always opt for whole milk
  - ○ Avoid commercial skim milk and dairy
- ➢ Eggs are excellent sources of powerful nutrients
  - ○ Pasture-raised is the best option
  - ○ "Cage-Free" and "Vegetarian-Fed" are simply marketing terms

6. The Calorie Myth

Buzzwords are powerful. Often times when a buzzword catches on it spreads like wildfire. There is no better example than the buzzword **calorie**. We have become a society *obsessed* with calories. Everyone and their mother have decided to count them, most without the slightest clue as to what they are. Ask yourself; do you know what a calorie is?

I didn't know what they were until about two years ago when researching to write *Ketogenic Catastrophe*. Simply put, a calorie is a <u>unit of heat</u>. (1) It is the heat energy generated by a piece of food. To measure how many calories are in a particular food, you must **ignite** the food, then capture and measure the heat that was released. This heat is used to calculate the caloric value.

> **Example** - Let's say you want to find out how many calories are in a double bacon cheeseburger you are about to eat. To do this, first get a thermometer and hold it above that mouth-watering burger. Then you'll need to ignite the burger and measure the heat it emits. The HEAT emitted is measured and used to calculate calories. The more heat, the more calories. A single patty burger with no cheese will emit less heat than a double

bacon cheeseburger; therefore the double bacon burger has more calories. **Remember, calories are units of heat**.

This was an oversimplified example. The real measurement of calories takes place inside what is called a calorimeter, and very precise calculations are made to determine the real caloric value. (2) Modern technology has given us the ability to be very confident with these numbers. It's all very accurate. However, this accuracy means nothing if counting calories is meaningless to weight-loss!

This may sound a bit jarring if you believe the calories-in calories-out theory of weight-loss, which states weight-loss will occur by consuming fewer calories than your body uses, creating a calorie deficit. This "less calories equals more weight-loss" paradigm completely ignores how human digestion works. A basic understanding of the digestive system is the key to realizing the pointlessness of counting calories. Knowing the number of calories we consume could be useful in *some cases*, but as we will find out shortly, it is not the main determinant of weight-loss or overall wellbeing. As we explore the basics of human digestion, you will see how calorie content loses its importance in favor of other dietary factors, namely nutritional content.

HUMAN DIGESTION

Human digestion isn't all that hard to understand. In fact, it's easy. Digestion starts the moment you take a bite of that double bacon cheeseburger. Your teeth pulverize the burger as saliva begins the enzymatic process of breaking it down. Then the stomach and upper intestines break down and **absorb nutrients** from the burger, while the lower intestines dispose of the waste. Accessory organs to digestion include the pancreas, liver, and gallbladder, each serving their function to help your body **absorb nutrients**.

In 100 lifetimes you could not count the number of bacteria that reside in your gastrointestinal tract. This bacterium is the main driver of digestion, supported by different enzymes and bile which help facilitate the breakdown and absorption process. Amazingly, food can be in transit for several days and travel up to 30ft as it moves through the GI tract. About an hour after you eat, food arrives in the small intestine where most digestion takes place. Next stop is the large intestine where digestible food is fermented by the gut flora. The waste is then expelled after digestion has finished, sometimes in a horrific display of sound and smell.

As this food is broken down and moves through your digestive system, the **nutrients** within the food are **extracted** and converted to energy which allows your body to function. Without these nutrients, you are dead. This is the main purpose of human digestion: to extract the necessary "fuel" to power your body. Proteins, carbohydrates, lipids (fat), vitamins, minerals, and many enzymes are the **fuel your body needs**. (3)

This begs the question; what does a calorimeter have to do with your body absorbing the fuel it needs? As you recall, the calorimeter **ignites** food to measure it, while your digestive system **breaks down** and absorbs the food we eat. In fact, when comparing human digestion to the calorimeter, very few similarities are found. At no time during human digestion is anything ever ignited. You will never burp smoke after eating a cheeseburger. Indigestion is not a small fire in your stomach, and it is most certainly not *literal* when someone says "my ass was on fire this morning from that spicy burrito last night." *Spicy chilies do not literally burn, they figuratively burn.* The calorimeter literally burns the food, your digestive system figuratively burns it. The waste product of the calorimeter is a pile of ash while the waste product of human digestion is a pile of...shit.

The biggest shortfall of the calorimeter is its inability to determine the nutritional value of food. It will not tell you how many vitamins and minerals the food has. It will not tell you the fat or protein content. And worst of all, it does not warn you of any harmful contaminants. Its only function is to measure the transfer of heat. Vitamin and mineral content **are not considered**.

To really hammer this home, let's consider another cheeseburger example. If you are on a 1500 calorie diet and a cheeseburger has 500 calories, you can eat three cheeseburgers per day, right? But what happens if you sprinkle a little rat poison on your second burger? The caloric level may not change so you should be ok to eat it, right? Of course not! Why? Because what really matters is the **nutritional profile** of the cheeseburger, not the calories. Adding rat poison may not change its calories, but it certainly changes its nutritional profile. The burger could still be 500 calories with rat poison added to it, but it will react very differently inside your body.

Here's another fun fact: Anything can have calories. Go grab a tissue, blow your nose, and put the used paper into a calorimeter and it will tell you how many calories it has. Do you care? Of course not. No one cares how many calories are in a used napkin. A piece of dog poop, an old running shoe, even that air freshener in your car will have calories, but those calories mean nothing. Why? Because you judge the dog poop on how easy it is to pick up, the running shoe on its comfort, and the air freshener on the smell it emits.

And so it goes with food. *Eat Fat, Get Fit* encourages you to judge food by its **nutritional profile**, not simply caloric value. Calories tell only a small part of your foods story. Choosing food based on calories is similar to choosing based on shape. Shape is a <u>descriptive</u> part of the food, like calories, but means nothing when evaluating its healthiness. An apple is not healthy because it is round. Why? Because the shape is not important. What really matters is the ***contents*** of the shape. Similarly, calories are not important, the **content** of the calories is what's important.

As you move forward with *Eat Fat, Get Fit* remember that human digestion is based on **nutrient absorption**. It functions by gathering vitamins, minerals, fat, protein, and carbohydrates (amongst other things) to be broken down and used as energy for your working body and mind. "Burning calories" is somewhat of a myth. They are not literally "burnt" as with the calorimeter. As you begin to remove foods with harmful

contaminants and increase your fat intake you will see a whole new world

of fitness open up before you. When you no longer worry about calories,

eating becomes much simpler, with less variables to think about. Eating

gets easier, and the easier a task, the more likely you are to succeed at it.

COUNT CHEMICALS NOT CALORIES

Do yourself an enormous favor: stop counting calories and start

counting chemicals. Chemical contamination is another reason for your

body to store fat. As a protection mechanism, your body will create fat

cells to store toxins (pesticides, insecticides, herbicides, fungicides, etc) in

order to keep them from your vital organs. This is why eating organic

fruits and veggies is so important for weight-loss & peak physical

performance. Many common agricultural chemicals have been shown to

promote chronic diseases such as cancer and heart disease. Also,

neurological disorders can be exacerbated, or possibly created, by long-

term exposure to harmful chemicals.

So where does this leave us? *Calories are overrated.* They could

be useful to monitor if weight-loss has stalled even after implementing

the other principles of *Eat Fat, Get Fit*, but this is unlikely. 99% of those looking for weight-loss and physical fitness can achieve their goals

without ever worrying about a calorie. In fact, when eating clean and

nutritious foods, calories can be seen as a good thing! They represent the

energy your body needs to continue functioning. Count them if you wish,

but remember, counting chemicals should always be your first priority.

KEY POINTS

- ➢ Calories are merely units of heat
- ➢ Calories do not consider nutritional content
- ➢ Rat poison is low in calories
- ➢ Human digestion uses bacteria, enzymes and acidic goo's to extract nutrients from food
  - ○ NOTHING IS EVER LITERALLY "BURNED"
- ➢ Counting chemicals instead of calories will ultimately help you lose weight and feel great

PART III: FAT AND FITNESS

From a performance enhancement point of view,
ketones (fat) function as an alternative fuel for your
brain and for your muscles. We are looking at the
application of a ketogenic diet and also supplemental
ketones to enhance cognitive performance and also
physical performance.

-Dr. Dominic D'Agostino

7. A Personal Weight-Loss Story

Back in 2009, my beer-belly had reached its peak. I was drinking and eating junk food regularly; the two main ingredients of the bulging midsection. I remember the day I finally made the decision to lose weight. It was summer of 2008, I was washing my car in front of the garage, and my roommate came out to have a beer with me while I layered the wax. I'll never forget the moment I bent over to wax the bottom side skirt, painfully aware my beer-belly was hanging out, and my roommate yelped; "Yea buddy! Look at that belly hang! Sexxxaaay!" I know he was just joking around, but I was immature and self-conscious at that point in my life, and it cut me to the core. I distinctly remember that being the day I decided to actually *try* to lose weight instead of just talking and thinking about it.

What followed that day were several attempts and failures in losing weight. Running 10-15 miles a week plus vigorous gym exercise was my starting point. After months of extreme effort I learned two things:

Number #1 - You can't outrun your fork. You can try, really, really hard. And it may seem like its working, but it's simply unsustainable. The amount of time and energy it takes to exercise enough to offset poor eating habits is simply too much in the long run. You will get tired, you will feel like crap, and you will likely give up. Trying to outrun your fork carries a 95% failure rate.

Number #2 - You can't outrun the beer. See above, replace "poor eating habits" with "excessive beer drinking."

After exercise failed, my next approach was a low-fat diet. Fruit and veggie smoothies with fat-free milk alternatives were the latest craze. A grilled chicken breast with steamed veggies became a normal meal. When combined with exercise this seemed to help, but progress was slow, and often stalled. I later realized this was likely due to fat **cravings** which caused me to cheat and eat the wrong things. These emotional triggers, as we will learn in Chapter 14, can be difficult to overcome.

Finally, in 2013, I came across research which claimed increasing fat intake while cutting down on carbs will increase weight-loss. I was captivated by this seemingly contradictory claim and buried myself in reading about it. After enough research, I decided to give it a shot. I was not prepared for what happened next. In dramatic fashion, within in a span of only six months, my wife and I each shed 30lbs of fat! To be honest, I didn't think I had 30lbs to lose. After my extraordinary weight-loss several people privately asked me if I was starving myself or on drugs! Interestingly enough, I was eating more than ever.

It's was very empowering to know what was actually happening to my body. The food I ate was literally sending signals which determined my metabolism. When I ate a large amount of sugar, my body had to release a larger amount of insulin to bring blood sugar back down. When in the blood, insulin signals the body to store fat. (1) When my caveman ancestor came across an abundant source of sugar (honey, fruit, etc), his body recognized this as a high-value source of energy, and converted excess glucose to fat for later use. It made perfect sense. For modern me on the other hand, spiking my blood sugar daily with donuts, pizza, pasta, sodas, and beer, this was not good.

The occasional jackpot of fruit or honey turned into daily blasts of sugar from candy, soda, and doughnuts. My life was consumed with refined carbohydrates. I think back to all the ice cream and candy I ate; all the pizzas and soda. It makes perfect sense as to why I had a beer-belly.

No question. What was once an occasional insulin spike had become a daily routine.

For years my glucose and insulin levels were spiking out of control, and my body was constantly in fat-storage mode. I was in a negative feedback loop. Eat sugar, make insulin, store fat. Eat sugar, make insulin, store fat. Over and over and over again. Once I decreased sugar and increased fat, my life changed dramatically. I've been lean for three years now, with no sign of going back. *Eat Fat, Get Fit* is my account of success. It is the path I took to the six-pack I have today. Not everyone will react the same way, and to those who don't I wish you good luck in finding your right path. The vast majority of you will succeed if you can simply stick with it. Give it time, give it practice, and always remember to keep pushing forward. You must learn to love the grind.

KEY POINTS

- ➢ **Avoiding fat cravings will increase the likelihood of cheat meals**
- ➢ **Increased fat intake coincides with increased weight-loss**
  - ○ **The more dietary fat available the less fat storage your body will need**

- ➢ Insulin sends signals to the body to STORE FAT
- ➢ Carbohydrate consumption triggers insulin production
  - ○ <u>This is how sugar makes you fat</u>
- ➢ You body will naturally try and maintain a balanced state using whatever inputs you are giving it
  - ○ Your dietary choices affect its metabolic decisions

8. Sugar vs. Fat - The Energy Showdown

There's a war being waged this very moment inside your body. The two main energy companies which supply fuel to your body are in deep conflict. The "glucose factory," which uses sugar, carbohydrate, glycogen, or protein to create energy, is clearly the bigger organization. They control the majority of energy production for your body, and they like it that way. The "fat-factory," which utilizes ketones from fat for energy, doesn't agree with this. For years they've complained about their lack of contribution to your energy needs. They are fed up, and want their fair share of the energy pie.

In its simplest form, food is the fuel these energy companies use. To get that fuel into the factories, your digestive system must first break down what you eat and extract the raw materials needed by each factory. These raw materials are used to create the energy needed to keep you moving and thinking all day. As long as the raw materials are being supplied, you will have energy to write emails, talk on the phone, lift boxes, etc, etc. These factories are always at work.

The glucose factory is excellent at providing instant energy. For high intensity exercises such as heavy lifting or sprinting, they are the best at providing immediate energy. The explosive and instant nature of the glucose factory makes it a perfect fit for these tasks. However, they may not be so great for things like sitting at your desk or couch. Think of using jet fuel for your minivan. It's over kill. It can cause long-term damage to your car.

Relying exclusively on your glucose factory for energy has its limitations. First off, your liver can only store a small amount of glycogen (glucose) for energy; generally about 1500 calories worth. Once this stored glucose is depleted, often in a matter of a few hours, you will need to consume more glucose before hypoglycemia (weakness, clumsiness, shakiness, trouble thinking, confusion, irritation, headache, etc) sets in. (1) Most of the time this isn't a problem because glucose is available almost anywhere. A piece of candy or a granola bar will stop hypoglycemic symptoms immediately. This becomes a fine line to walk, and if you find yourself in a situation without food for several hours, your journey will become difficult, and frustrating.

The next drawback is what's called the "glucose rollercoaster." Eating glucose raises your blood sugar and you feel energized; *"Yeah let's do this, I love my job!"* Then, elevated blood sugar triggers the release of insulin into your blood, which reduces blood sugar and causes fatigue; *"My job sucks and so do you, I'm starving!"* To regain energy you must eat additional glucose; *"Hell-Ya! Let's do this!"* which then releases insulin, reduces blood sugar and causes low energy and hunger; *"Screw this, I'm tired!"* This cycle will repeat itself until you make your way to bed. The glucose factory has most of us stuck on this daily rollercoaster. Why? <u>Because it's normal</u>. In our society, sugar-burning has become the norm. And not just normal, but also incredibly easy. So easy in fact anyone can do it.

The fat-factory works a bit differently than its glucose counterpart. While the glucose factory relies on sugar, carbohydrate, or protein, the fat-factory runs on fat, or ketones. Both factories can produce adequate power to fuel the body, but their efficiency levels are much different. In fact, where the glucose factory struggles, the fat-factory excels. This can be seen clearly when comparing each factory's ability to store energy. The glucose factory can store around 1,500 calories of usable energy in the form of glucose, while the fat factory can store around **100,000 calories** of usable energy in the form of fat. Even an extremely lean athlete will have several days' worth of energy stored as fat on their body.

When the fat-factory is given more responsibility for your energetic needs you'll notice several "side effects" that sound more like miracles. For example, you will be able to go longer between meals while still maintaining plenty of energy. To test the limits of this, my friend Gabe and I decided to try a 3-day fast. No food, no coffee, nothing, only water with sea salt in the mornings. To be clear, both of us are extremely fat-adapted, meaning our fat-factories have a much larger share of the energy pie. You should never attempt a fast unless you have cultivated this ability in yourself first. We will learn more about fat-adaption in the next chapter.

I was a bit nervous before starting since I had never gone more than a day without eating up to that point in my life. I thought for sure I would get cranky, tired, a headache, and want to give up on the 2nd day. To my complete shock, three days breezed by without a problem and I felt better than ever. Before breaking the fast, Gabe and I went to the gym and preformed dead-lifts, an exercise involving lifting dead-weight off the ground. We did not experience the crash many athletes face, often called "bonking," and we both felt an overwhelming sense of euphoria. The fat-factory has an impressive supply of stored energy that is available to the body even without eating. The test was successful, and we have now incorporated a quarterly 3-day fast into our lives.

Another benefit of the fat-factory managing your energy levels is the absence of the notorious glucose rollercoaster. Think about it; your entire life has been spent on a roller coaster at Disneyland. Up-and-down, up-and-down. All day every day. Imagine waking up late for work and don't have time to eat breakfast, and your last meal was over 10 hours ago at dinner. You get to work and are slammed with calls and people demanding answers from you, so you may have to take a late lunch. Can you imagine the glucose factory workers panicking as you're about to run out of fuel? You can actually *feel* that panic in the form of anxiety about when your next meal will be.

If your fat-factory is working as it should (meaning you are fat-adapted), then you will be able to make it to lunch. The near vertical rollercoaster drop never happens. Your metabolism will simply switch to your fat-factory for energy and you can carry on with your day. **Having this ability is an incredible asset**. The process of burning fat instead of glucose for energy is called ketosis. (2) To use a car analogy, if a regular gas burning car is a sugar-burner, then a fancy new electric car is a fat-burner. Both cars are able to get from point-A to point-B, they simply use different fuel sources.

Ideally we want to be somewhere in the middle of a fat-burner and sugar-burner, or what I've termed a hybrid. A hybrid metabolism can switch between glucose and fat based on what's available and best for the situation. This does not happen overnight and takes work to achieve. *Eat Fat, Get* Fit will give you this ability if you stick with it. Having the ability to use both sources of fuel makes your human vehicle much more flexible, and as we know, the most successful people at anything are also the most flexible.

The days of the glucose factory are numbered as more and more people wake up to the wonderful world of burning fat for energy. Eating more fat will turbocharge your weight-loss, increase physical performance, and improve mental cognition. The next step is to become *fat-adapted*.

KEY POINTS

> **Glucose (sugar) is the most common type of fuel used today**
>> ○ **The glucose factory**

- ➤ The body can store very limited amounts of glucose for future use
- ➤ Hypoglycemia occurs when the glucose factory runs out of glucose
  - ○ Emotional instability, headache, fatigue, dizziness, anxiety, etc.
- ➤ The human body is actually designed to burn fat more efficiently
  - ○ The fat-factory
- ➤ The fat-factory can store 100,000 calories worth of energy on the body
  - ○ Sugar is usually depleted in a matter of hours
- ➤ A "hybrid" can transition between sugar and glucose as necessary
  - ○ This is called metabolic flexibility

9. Becoming Fat-Adapted

Being fat-adapted is exactly what it sounds like; your body is adapted to fat. Most everyone is capable of this because we all share the same basic digestion and metabolism. The rate at which most people become fat-adapted follows a very predictable, exponential curve. Like a locomotive at a standstill, your body's fat burning abilities are at a standstill. Your fat-factory's gears are not moving. This is the bottom of the curve. Most of us are stagnating, locked in the dogma of low-fat, high-carb diet recommendations and fear of heart disease and obesity. We are *stuck* as sugar-burners. The process of fat-adaption begins with a few simple steps which generate the momentum needed get your fat-factory operating effectively.

When fully fat-adapted, your body has the ability to burn fat for **submaximal** energy needs, meaning anything less than full physical exertion. Glucose is "spared" in favor of fat. In order to become fat-adapted, the first step is to limit glucose. As glucose is limited, your body will have no choice but to use fat for fuel. Be warned, the glucose factory may react very stubbornly to your attempt at becoming fat-adapted, and this could be the hardest part of the whole process! If your body is comfortable burning glucose, any significant restriction can trigger a hypoglycemic (low blood glucose) response. You will be hungry, cranky, and fatigued. It will not be fun. Slowly increasing fat while slowing decreasing carbohydrate will allow you to become fat-adapted and avoid hypoglycemic symptoms. The idea is to spread this process out over several weeks.

Increasing dietary fat too quickly can cause loosening of the stool, also called "disaster pants." The name is more of a joke since you won't actually crap your pants, you'll just need to find a bathroom rather quickly. Your digestive system is unable to keep up with the demand of so much fat so early in your journey. Once your system is accustomed to metabolizing more fat, then you can increase the amount until you find your comfort zone. (1)

FIND FAT OPPORTUNITIES

When increasing fat, start first by locating areas within your diet you can increase fat intake. Coffee is a perfect example that many people use as a stepping stone. Adding a tablespoon of coconut oil or grass-fed butter to coffee in the morning is a great way to increase fat intake; and it tastes delicious! Simply add virgin coconut oil or grass-fed butter to your coffee and blend it up. Fat-blended coffee has become all the rage throughout Silicon Valley. High performing tech CEOs and entrepreneurs have been using this method for years. Made popular by Dave Asprey of www.bulletproofexec.com, "Bulletproof Coffee" involves blending grass-fed butter and MCT oil in with coffee. This coffee has become one of the hottest trends amongst the countries top athletes and executives.

WARNING If your goal is weight-loss you must be sure to decrease sugar intake at the same time you increase fat. If you simply add more fat while continuing to consume high levels of sugar (sugary drinks, candy, pastries, etc) you will likely GAIN weight. Obviously you are not here for advice on *adding* body fat.

Cooking with butter, ghee, or lard are other excellent ways to increase fat. Add olive oil to your salad, bacon to your breakfast, or avocado to your lunch. Honestly, put avocado on everything. Eggs with avocado and potatoes in the morning, on a sandwich for lunch, on top of soups or roasts, and even in smoothies. Avocado goes on everything. Find a source of fat that is enjoyable then see how many places you can incorporate it.

The smoothie, which is an excellent tool for weight-loss, has become a beacon of hope for those struggling to shed excess pounds.

However, the struggling dieter often misses the most important ingredient; FAT! The high-fat smoothie is a nutritional powerhouse and a powerful appetite suppressor. The smoothie can be your best friend if used properly. Try starting your day with a high-fat option of your favorite smoothie and tweak it as you go. An avocado provides an excellent base for creaminess, while a banana and other fruit will add needed sweetness. The smoothie is also an excellent way to sneak in veggies without the annoying part of having to chew them up and taste them. Nuts and seeds can also add beneficial nutrients and fat. Finish with a liquid base of full-fat milk or even a milk substitute, such as full-fat coconut milk (a great alternative to dairy), or almond milk.

A tablespoon or two of coconut oil or grass-fed butter can kick the fat content up if needed. The goal of the smoothie is to completely nourish your body and curb those pesky hunger pangs. The absence of hunger will allow you to perform at work without succumbing to the dreaded mid-morning sweets craving. Those doughnuts sitting in your office won't look nearly as appealing after you've had a powerful high-fat smoothie for breakfast. This stage of fat-adaption is often where people give up, because the results haven't yet poured in as the fat-factory is still ramping up production.

Here's a quick beginners recipe that will get you going in the right direction. Remember to use enough liquid. Gulping down an overly thick smoothie is not fun. A sweetener like Xylitol can be used if extra sweetness is needed. Play with the ratios and ingredients until you find something you enjoy!

Ingredients:

- 1 banana
- ½ cup frozen blueberries/other berries (organic)
- 1 small avocado
- 1 handful spinach (organic)
- 2 tbls chia seeds
- 1-2 tsp cinnamon
- 1-2 tbls virgin coconut oil
- 1-2 tbls raw nuts or nut butter (cashew, almond, pecan, etc)

Base (choose 1 or 2):

- Whole grass-fed milk (8-12oz)
- Coconut milk (1/2 can + water)
- Organic almond milk
- Water

Fat-adaption is crucial to the *Eat Fat, Get Fit* approach. Once you develop the ability to efficiently metabolize fat, you will find yourself in a new world of dietary options. The reality of having only butter and coffee for breakfast, then nothing else until a late lunch, or even dinner, is awaiting you. This will take several weeks to months of slow increases before you can attempt such meal schedules. Slow and steady is the best approach and will produce the most desired results.

KEY POINTS

- ➢ Becoming fat-adapted involves a slow transition to increased dietary fat
  - ○ Going too quickly can spell "disaster-pants"
- ➢ Your digestive system must "ramp-up" its ability to efficiently metabolize high quantities of fat
- ➢ Cold-pressed coconut oil and grass-fed butter are excellent fat starting points
- ➢ Smoothies are a quick and easy way to increase healthy fat intake
  - ○ Xylitol can be used to increase sweetness

10. A New World of Physical Fitness

Fitness is easy when following the *Eat Fat, Get* Fit program. This is because only about 10% of the fitness results most people desire come from exercise done at the gym, while the other 90% comes from the effort put into the kitchen! Imagine all the time, energy, and resources spent at the gym with a personal trainer, only to receive 10% of the results you desire! This is not an effective use of your time. If your goal is simply to look good naked, following the dietary recommendations provided in this book is essentially all most people will need to do.

For those who wish to push the limits of their body, eating more fat has been shown to produce almost unbelievable results in the area of sports performance. Athletes around the world have caught wind of the amazing benefits of increasing dietary fat. When paired with strength and endurance training, high-fat diets have catapulted competitors ahead of their rivals. This new paradigm in strength training has gained momentum with seasoned pros like Dr. Dominic D'Agostino blazing the trail ahead. Dr. D'Agostino, who dabbles in power lifting and cancer research, was able to dead-lift 500lbs after fasting for 7 days! For more info from Dr. D'Agostino, visit his site www.ketonutrition.org.

Inflammation is the enemy of performance. Low-carb/high-fat diets are inherently anti-inflammatory, which means they *reduce* oxidative stress during exercise. Lactic acid buildup is greatly reduced which helps the body recover faster between workouts. (1) What was once a glucose game is quickly becoming a fat dominated arena. Below is an excerpt from an Ohio State News Room release titled "Elite performance on diet with minimal carbs represents paradigm shift in sports nutrition":

> *"Elite endurance athletes who eat very few carbohydrates burned more than twice as much fat as high-carb athletes during maximum exertion and prolonged exercise in a new study – the highest fat-burning rates under these conditions ever seen by researchers."* (2)

So what are today's most high performing endurance athletes doing that is changing the face of physical competition? A perfect example are the marathon runners who follows a low-carb, high-fat diet. Until recently, marathon runners relied heavily on glucose to fuel their bodies through the grueling 26.2 mile run. The night before a marathon, runners notoriously "carb-loaded" with a giant plate of pasta and bread to ensure maximum glucose was available as fuel. However, since the body can only store about 1500 calories of glucose in the form of glycogen, this approach has obvious weaknesses. Throughout the race, sugary sports drinks and glucose supplements must be handed out to exhausted runners, without which these runners would simply <u>run out of energy</u>...pun intended. The new breed of runner understands the body is able to store much more energy in the form of fat. Even an extremely lean athlete will have several days' worth of energy stored as fat on their body. These new-age runners can slurp down MCT oil instead of sugar and maintain optimal energy levels throughout the race.

As mentioned earlier, a friend of mine and I completed a 3-day fast. That's 72hrs with <u>no food</u>. At the end of the third day we went to the gym and performed deadlifts. My blood sugar had bottomed out at 32 the second day and remained in the 30's until the fast was broken. During our workout my blood ketone levels reached 6.6mm/L. Levels this high have been shown in multiple studies to be effective at combating cancer, epilepsy, diabetes, and other chronic degenerative diseases. (3,4)

During the workout neither of us bonked (ran out of glucose) as most athletes would. There was no fainting, feeling sick, or any other negative side effect. Our bodies operated exactly as nature intended. If you can imagine a day before grocery stores, sometimes humans went several days without food. This was actually a normal part of life. When food isn't available, and the body is properly "fat-adapted," your metabolism will turn to ketones instead of glucose. This is Mother Nature at work. We live in a society where sugar, in the form of carbohydrates, is available everywhere we go. There is never a biological *need* for our metabolism to switch into fat-burning mode.

Once fat-adapted you will notice exercise gets easier. Even more amazing is that you can workout LESS and get in better shape! *"Abs are made in the kitchen"* is a popular phrase in the ketogenic diet community. In fact, you can do almost zero exercise and still shed weight at alarming rates if you really focus on following the *Eat Fat, Get Fit* dietary principles. However, if you skip exercise you will also miss out on many benefits that come along with it, namely mental clarity, increased endorphin production, and the feeling of accomplishment after a workout is completed. (5) Many gym-goers (including myself) consider the mental benefits of exercise to be the most rewarding aspect, while the physical results are a sort of "icing on the cake."

Whether you desire maximum physical performance or simply want that summer body you've always wanted, eating more fat and less sugar is the way to go. High-fat endurance athletes have taken the competitive world by storm while busy moms drop the dreaded baby weight and are rushing out to buy new bikinis. These possibilities can become reality sooner than you can imagine. All that's needed is for you to decide it's time to make the necessary changes. After you make that decision, your life will change in ways you never thought possible!

KEY POINTS

- Performance athletes are beginning to use *Eat Fat, Get Fit* principles to propel themselves ahead of the competition
- Marathon runners currently rely heavily on glucose
    - Ketogenic runners rely on fat and perform with greater efficiency
- Exercise becomes easier when your body can utilize fat for energy production
- Having clear physical goals will help you achieve them
- Exercise produces mental clarity

11. Get Smart and Sexy - How Fat Improves Cognition

Do you ever feel a bit...*hazy?* Sort of like walking through fog. How about *scattered?* How would you rate your current ability to focus or concentrate? If you feel you could use some improvement in these areas, you are in luck. The *Eat Fat, Get Fit* approach has a few other "side-effects" that many believe to be even more powerful than the ability to give you that rockin' bikini-bod or a shredded 6-pak.

For years experts have claimed glucose is the brain's main source of fuel. And guess what, they are right. *"Glucose is virtually the sole fuel for the human brain, except during prolonged starvation. The brain lacks fuel stores and hence requires a continuous supply of glucose. It consumes about 120g daily, accounting for some 60% of the utilization of glucose by the whole body in the resting state." (1)* So we know the brain uses glucose. A lot of it. But we aren't here to talk about the brain running on glucose, we are here to talk about it running on fat. First, let's find out if the brain is even capable of doing such a thing. The following is from the conclusion of a study published on the National Institutes of Health (NIH) website:

*"These data are consistent with our previous studies that, in combination with increased ketosis and increased transport of ketone bodies at the blood brain barrier, there are more ketones available for **brain metabolism**."* (2)

So the brain can certainly run on fat. Now, let's ask the **million dollar question**; the question on everyone's mind. If this were a gameshow, the cameras would be zoomed in as Regis Philbin slowly grabs the white card and asks:

"Which energy source fuels the brain with better efficiency: Sugar or Fat?"

The audience is silent. Tension in the room is so thick you could cut it with a knife. The time is now to give an answer! Let's have it!?! **SUGAR OR FAT?**

Not only will eating more fat and less sugar make you more physically fit, but it will also make you more MENTALLY fit. Energy levels increase while fogginess dramatically decreases. People who eat more fat and less sugar report razor sharp focus with an almost superhuman ability to concentrate for extended periods of time. High-powered executives and tech startup entrepreneurs alike are leveraging the benefits of fat metabolism in the brain to unleash hurricane levels of cognitive performance. The brain-power tides are changing.

If you recall the story from Chapter 10 about my 3-day fast, I was able to perform physically at a very high level, but you didn't get the *full* story. My mental clarity was also through the roof. While we fasted Monday thru Wednesday, and I also went to work, cooked dinner for my family, and worked on my previous book at night. I felt unstoppable. At one point I measured blood ketone levels at 6.6mM/L, meaning glucose usage in the brain could have been down 66%, maybe more. My blood sugar was in the 30's during day two and three of the fast, and I felt as if I was taking some sort of mental performance enhancer. Fat metabolism in the brain is no joke!

Dr. David Perlmutter's book *Grain Brain* is an absolute must read for those who wish to dig deeper into how the brain functions on fat. Dr. Perlmutter claims carbohydrates actually <u>cause</u> brain aging while fat <u>prevents</u> it. An epidemic of dementia has exploded across the country and very few people seem to understand why. Some experts have even begun to refer to these symptoms as type-3 diabetes. A study performed by the Mayo Clinic found that test subjects who consumed large quantities of carbs quadrupled their risk of pre-dementia, aka "mild cognitive impairment." (3,4) Interestingly, a mediterrarian style diet was shown to slow or prevent similar cognitive decline. (5) The *Eat Fat, Get Fit* approach contains principles of a mediterrarian style diet, namely healthy fat from oils and lots of veggies.

High-fat diets have been shown to reduce inflammation, which can improve your mental performance. Inflammation in the brain can reduce cognitive capabilities and leave you *thinking* slower. Do you wish to think slower? I didn't think so. Your brain is a major target for inflammation, so we must be vigilant in protecting it.

So, can eating more fat really make you smarter? Absolutely. The mental performance gains that accompany increased fat intake are unrivaled. From personal experience I can report this to be true, and many others continue to verify this claim daily. Only some sort of smart-drug can match these results. In the next section, we will lay the groundwork for the *Eat Fat, Get Fit* game plan and explore several lifestyle roadblocks that await you. You'll be given a mental framework for success that will ultimately lead to your weight-loss goals.

KEY POINTS

- The brain can operate on both glucose AND ketones
- Brain-fog or haziness can actually be a symptom of glucose overload in the brain
  - Pre-dementia is being dubbed type-3 diabetes
- Reports of increased cognitive abilities from people in ketosis are extremely common
  - From personal experience I can vouch for this
- High-fat diets reduce inflammation

PART IV: EAT FAT, GET FIT GAME PLAN

"Energy and persistence conquer all things"

- Benjamin Franklin

12. Home Field Advantage

Every athlete knows how important the home field advantage is. Being on your home turf, when faced with any challenge, has been shown to be extremely beneficial. The crowd is on your side, you have a more intimate connection to the field, and you will never struggle with finding your way around. Your home field is where you will perform best, and statistics will verify this.

Similarly, it is at your home field where your diet will perform its best. Cooking meals at home is of utmost importance when following the *Eat Fat, Get Fit* program. Your home is a place of safety and control. You are not at the whim of someone else's decisions or preferences when refueling your body. Failing to take full advantage of the home field is the #1 reason for failure in weight-loss and physical fitness. The following are helpful concepts and frameworks to use as you enter into this new phase of your life.

COOK ONCE, EAT TWICE

Hell, eat three times if you can. Preparing large meals that ensure leftovers is one of the most important practices for those who lead busy lives. Cook once, eat twice, has been the backbone of my family's dietary strategy as both my wife and I work full time. Tomorrow's lunch is almost always leftovers from the night before. This strategy will also pay huge dividends to your pocketbook. If you frequently buy lunch, you could save upwards of $2,000 per year per person by bringing food from home. Make sure to have adequate storage containers, preferable glass/Pyrex.

LOVE YOUR SLOW-COOKER

If you don't already, learn to love your slow-cooker. If you don't have one, spend the money and get one. To successfully follow *Eat Fat, Get Fit* you must spend more time prepping and cooking your own food. The slow-cooker is an excellent tool that allows you to simply toss a bunch of food into a pot and walk away. Eight hours later, when you return home from work, you have a complete meal waiting for you. There are wonderful slow-cooker recipe books out there that will guide you through this. Get yourself a Paleo slow-cooker recipe book and finding a few favorites from there.

Example Recipe:

3 pound grass-fed brisket
4 chopped carrots
2 chopped sweet potatoes
1 chopped onion
1 head chopped cabbage
5 garlic cloves
4 tbls sea salt
½ tsp black pepper & cumin

2 tbls grass-fed butter
Bone Broth

Directions: Season the brisket, and throw everything in the crock-pot, make sure the meat is submerged, cook on low for 8 hrs. Done.

MASTER THE SMOOTHIE

As we discussed earlier in the book, smoothies are an excellent tool for weight-loss and physical fitness. You can cram an unbelievable amount of nutritional value, including precious fats, into a portable and easy-to-consume meal. Everyone has different preferences when it comes to smoothies, so play with the ingredients and ratios to figure out what works best for you. Not surprisingly, many people find high-fat smoothies to be one of the most delicious meals they've ever had. It is difficult to find anything that compares to taste and feel of a power-packed fatty smoothie.

Example Recipe:

12oz grass-fed whole milk
1 banana
½ avocado
2 cups organic frozen berries
¼ cup goji berries
2 tbls coconut oil
2 tbls chia seeds
1 tbls almond butter
1 raw egg yolk (optional)

**Add water/ice if you want to play with the consistency

This smoothie packs a **powerful** nutritional punch. Those ingredients are chalked full of precious vitamins, minerals, and fatty goodness. Smoothies are also an easy way to cram more veggies into your day, which is always a good idea. Try adding a handful or two of organic spinach or chard. A raw egg yolk will increase creaminess and the nutritional quality of the smoothie. Try tossing in a chunk of a pre-cooked sweet potato to bring sweetness levels up if you desire. Need it sweeter? Use alternatives like Xylitol or raw honey instead of sugar.

If you want to make the best smoothies you'll want to invest in a high quality blender such as a BlendTec or Vitamix. The prices may *appear* to be high, but after owning a BlendTec for two years I can promise you they are worth every penny. You will be more likely to enjoy the smoothie if it is pureed and not chunky. Confidence in your home field will increase if you have the tools to make things run and blend smoothly.

SNACKS

Having snacks available is mandatory. How many times have you come home from work and just wanted to open the cupboard and grab something quick? It happens all the time. If you don't have a healthy option available you are likely to say: *"Screw it, I want some Cheetos right now and I don't care what Eric said in that book."* Always keep in mind, <u>the fewer ingredients the better</u>. If you check the ingredients list and find a bunch of words you cannot pronounce, it's probably not "food" you are eating, but rather something "food-like" as Dr. Alejandro Junger calls it.

Snack Ideas:
- Grass-fed cheese
- Nuts and seeds
- Grass-fed cottage cheese
- Apple or veggies w/ almond butter
- Organic hummus w/ veggies
- Chips (Boulder potato chips w/ three ingredients)
- Paleo or keto approved protein bars
- Organic dark chocolate
- Your favorite fruits or veggies

The main thing to remember is to keep your home field stocked with snacks you KNOW you will eat. It is pointless to have "healthy" options available if you will not touch them. Keep in mind finding healthy options you enjoy isn't hard. It may simply take trial-and-error until you find your match. Remember, every time you choose a healthy snack you have taken a step towards your goal instead of away from it. <u>These steps will compound into your desired results.</u>

SATISFY YOUR SWEET TOOTH

Simply denying your sweet tooth on your home turf is a rookie mistake. These emotional cravings can be stronger than most people realize, so having a game plan is important. The, *"I'm not going to eat sweet stuff anymore"* mindset is a recipe for failure. We must <u>understand</u> these cravings and be prepared for them BEFORE trying to cut back. This will greatly increase success rates.

<u>Dark chocolate</u> is a necessity for curbing the sugar cravings in our household. The cacao bean, from which dark chocolate is made, is packed full of antioxidants and good fats. Get yourself a stash of high quality dark chocolate so you are prepared for sweets cravings. Start low at 72% cacao and work your way up from there. Try dipping the dark chocolate in almond or peanut butter if you crave candy. My wife and I eat chocolate with almond butter nightly. It's the perfect desert with good fats to end the day.

Ripe bananas contain higher levels of sugar and work well to squash sugar cravings. The banana is nature's candy bar. Cover each bite with almond butter for a creamy treat. Craving dessert? A bowl of berries with coconut oil and raw pecans will also work wonders when craving dessert.

> **Dessert Bowl Ingredients:** Organic frozen blueberries, banana, coconut oil, pecans, cinnamon, dark chocolate.
>
> **Directions**: Slice the banana and combine with blueberries, pecans, and dark chocolate in a bowl. Drizzle 2tbls of coconut oil and add cinnamon to taste. Pretend its ice cream!

LEARN TO LOVE THE BOWL

Tortillas, buns, bread...these are all "vehicles" for transporting the real food (meat, veggies, and grains) into your mouth. They have become a part of our fast-paced culture, allowing the busiest of people to grab a meal to go. If you really want to turbocharge your weight-loss, throw everything into a bowl and skip the "food vehicles."

> **The Burger Bowl Ingredients:** One pound grass-fed ground beef (makes 4 patties), 2 sweet potatoes, lettuce, tomato, avocado, onion, organic ketchup and mustard, sauerkraut.
>
> **Directions**: Make a burger as you normally would, except leave out the bun and add everything to a bowl. Sweet potato fries pair perfectly with this meal. Use moderation with condiments like

ketchup as they often contain high amounts of added sugar. Mustard is an excellent low-sugar condiment. *Feeds 4, no leftovers*

The Burrito Bowl Ingredients: One pound grass-fed ground beef or organic chicken, 2 cups white rice, tomato paste, lettuce, tomato, onion, avocado, Mexican seasoning, cilantro, lime, sea salt

Directions: Make 2 cups of white rice, adding tomato sauce, garlic, and onion prior to cooking. In a pan, brown ground beef or chicken with onions and Mexican seasoning. Dump contents of pan (including fat) into the finished rice and mix. Add rice to a bowl with lettuce, tomato, avocado, lime, sea salt, and your favorite hot sauce. *Feeds 4, no leftovers*

The Chicken Teriyaki Bowl - Ingredients: white rice, veggies, chicken thighs, coconut amino's teriyaki sauce, avocado, MCT oil, grass-fed butter, sea salt

Directions: Add 1 tbls grass-fed butter to rice before cooking. Chop chicken and veggies into bite sized pieces, season with sea salt, pepper, chili flakes, and cook in a pan with butter. Combine meat and veggies with rice, add sauce to taste. Keep sea salt nearby.

The bowl is your friend in the *Eat Fat, Get Fit* lifestyle. It's easy, reliable, portable, and allows for almost endless options. **Get creative with it**. Think of what you crave and figure out a way to put it into a bowl. If you *must* have pasta, get an organic quinoa or rice version. These pasta's provide a smooth transition away from more highly processed and heavily contaminated wheat pastas that currently fill store shelves.

HAVE FUN

You are embarking on one hell of a journey. It will be filled with ups and down, trials and tribulations, success and failure. The most important thing you can do throughout this journey is to have fun with it. Laugh at your mistakes. Take pride in your successes and forgive yourself for your failures. If you have a partner in this journey, encourage and support them. Make it fun. But always remember to take advantage of your home field!

For more recipes and food related information visit:

www.paleoplatform.com

KEY POINTS

- ➢ Take advantage of eating at home as much as possible
- ➢ Cook once, eat twice (or three times!)
- ➢ Use your slow cooker, it is a powerful tool for weight-loss
  - o Low effort high yield meals
- ➢ Smoothies are an easy way to pack in tons of nutrients
- ➢ Be sure you always have healthy snacks ready to eat
  - o This will prevent cheating due to lack of instant gratification
- ➢ Don't ignore your sweet tooth!
- ➢ Use a bowl for your meals as much as possible
  - o Bread, tortillas, and shells are simply vehicles for real food
- ➢ Have fun with your food!

13. What to Eat When You're Out

Having the home field advantage is always preferable, but what about those times you must eat outside of your home? What are the best options if you're out at a restaurant or fast-food joint? This chapter will provide several guidelines to follow that help minimize the damage from eating out.

The path to your goal weight will be filled with many steps forward and many steps backwards. "Two-steps forward, one step back" is a common route. The forward steps represent nights you ate healthy food from home, while "back-steps" symbolize fast-food for lunch, the beer and hotdog at the baseball game, or a nice pasta dinner on the town with that special someone. The following recommendations allow you to turn these back-steps into *half* or *quarter-steps* backwards, as opposed to a full step back. Over time, these half and quarter-steps produce dramatic results for your weight-loss efforts. Remember, weight-loss is a marathon not a sprint. Commit these recommendations to memory and dramatic results will follow.

It's lunch time on Wednesday and you have nothing to eat. Life got a little hectic and you didn't *"cook once, eat twice."* It happens. Your stomach has begun to growl and you know it's time to eat before the crankiness emerges. There are a couple fast-food joints not far from the office, but you are unsure of what to get. Consider the following:

1. **Meat, Veggies, Starch, Whole Grains** - Say it out loud with me: MEAT, VEGGIES, STARCH, GRAINS. Want to get a burrito? Get a burrito bowl. Craving carbs? Stick to rice or potatoes. Order meals that are meat, protein, and veggies only. They exist on most menus, all you need to do is look, or ask.

2. **Protein Style** - If you're getting a burger, order it protein style (wrapped in lettuce). Get a double burger since the lack of bread may leave you craving more food.

3. **Find a Bowl** - Look for restaurants that serve chicken or beef bowls. Meat, veggies, and rice served in a bowl is a better option than something loaded with bread. Avoid "breaded" things like chicken tenders, unless they are grilled. Add MCT oil to these bowls.

4. **Drink Water** - Soda is often hardest thing to give up, particularly with meals, but it must be done. Raspberry Iced Tea is also a sugary drink...sorry. These "healthy alternatives" often have just as much sugar as soda. Unsweetened tea with lemon is

acceptable. Sparkling water with lemon/lime doesn't satisfy the taste buds like a soda, but your liver and pancreas will breathe a sigh of relief if you stick to it. Keep this in mind: *the excess flab on your belly sure wants you to order a refreshing soda, and it will thank you by growing larger.*

5. **Grilled not Fried** - Always choose the grilled option over fried. The oils used for frying are the lowest in quality and come highly oxidized.

6. **Easy on the Condiments** - Condiments are sugar offenders. Ketchup is packed with sugar, which is the reason it tastes so good! Surprise. Specialty sauces touted as the main attraction of a dish (Ex - Cilantro pesto dipping sauce) are likely filled with sugar and contain low quality oils. Mustard is your best option as it contains the fewest ingredients and the least amount of sugar.

7. **Add MCT Oil** - This simple trick will allow you to boost the fat content of any meal. MCT oil is a clear, tasteless liquid that will make your food taste better! It's a sort of flavor enhancer. Put it on your chicken bowl, burger, or anything you order. MCT Oil will leave you feeling more fulfilled and allow you to maintain higher energy levels for the duration of the day.

8. **No dessert** - Keep an organic dark chocolate bar on hand if you are like me and crave sweets after a meal. Any dessert you order while out is going to work against you. Plan ahead for these situations if you think you will struggle.

It is impossible to go over every lunch scenario here, so you'll need to adapt as you run into things. Keep these basics in mind and you will make much progress over the coming weeks and months.

Now it's Friday evening, you worked hard all week and need a night out on the town. Maybe that means hanging out with friends, maybe with your spouse or kids, possibly even some nice alone time to help clear your mind. Whatever this means to you, it is important to remember that the *Eat Fat, Get Fit* game plan does not stay at home. It's like your wallet; you take it wherever you go. Here are a few more things to remember, and even a substitution for those looking to have some drinks:

1. **Avoid the bread** - Sorry, I had to say it again. Dinner is the hardest time to do this. Have you ever wondered why restaurants often bring out a basket of bread before anything else? It's cheap

filler that ultimately leaves you hungrier in a shorter span of time. Stay strong and pass on the bread basket.

2. **Banish the Beer** - Beer is a heavy offender to the *Eat Fat, Get Fit* program. As you transition to this new lifestyle your body needs time to reset and clear the junk out. Beer is simply liquid wheat and sugar. To be honest, it is almost impossible to know what's in your beer since 99% of them do not list their ingredients. Strangely enough it is one of the only foods/drinks NOT REQUIRED by law to list its ingredients. <u>We have no idea how much sugar or what preservatives are being added</u>. Instead of beer, try the following substitutions:

   a. Nor-Cal Margarita: agave tequila with soda water and fresh lime. This is your best option for booze.

   b. Potato vodka or Gin with non-sugary mixers work well also. These will also leave you less hung-over the following day.

3. **Avoid Pasta** - Italian restaurants can feel like a torture chamber when trying to *Eat Fat, Get Fit*. While pasta is delicious, we must remember it is a highly processed carbohydrate that will spike your blood sugar, thus spiking insulin, which signals the body to

store fat. This book is not called *Eat Carbs, Get Fat*. If you find yourself at an Italian joint, order something that contains only meat and veggies with potatoes or rice. Remember, the more you limit carbs (even potatoes and rice) the quicker you will shed excess body fat.

4. **Add MCT** - It's embarrassing to pull out a little container of MCT oil and dinner if you are with other people. If you can get over it, do it. If not, just do this when you are alone or with family.

I imagine about half the readers of this book just clicked delete or threw their copy in the nearest fireplace. By far, beer and pasta carry the largest emotional connections. Why? They make us *feel good*. Almost nothing *feels* better than a giant plate of pasta with some buttery garlic bread and a tasty beer. Carbs on carbs on carbs. So remember, and say it with me if necessary: MEAT, VEGGIES, & STARCH. These are your target foods when eating out. In the next chapter we will dig into the emotional connections we have to foods and find ways to overcome them for good.

KEY POINTS

- ➤ **Avoid bread**
- ➤ **Drink water, unsweetened tea, or sparkling water**
- ➤ **Ask for grilled instead of fried**

- ➤ Meat - Veggies - Fruit - Grains - Starch
  - ○ Target these foods only
- ➤ Easy on the condiments, they are often hidden sources of sugar
- ➤ Skip dessert
- ➤ Avoid beer and pasta

14. Big Fat Emotions

Whether we admit it or not, emotions influence much of our daily lives. In fact, most of what we think and do is a product of our emotional state. In my early stages of weight-loss I struggled greatly with emotional attachments to food. What made it so difficult was that I didn't fully understand what was happening, so I found myself in various negative feedback loops that stunted my progress. By understanding these various knee-jerk type emotional reactions that arise in our lives we will be better equipped to face the many challenges that await us.

In order to give you a clearer picture of how our emotional reactions operate, I'd like to tell you a story about Joe, a man who walks to work. This story will help you to understand the learning curve involved with overcoming emotional food cravings.

Joe was walking to work on Monday and fell into a manhole. After falling, he had no idea what happened. Confused and frustrated, it took him hours to figure out how to get out of the sewer, and when he finally did, he swore he'd never let it happen again. On Tuesday, the same thing happened. Joe was walking down the street, minding his own business, and BAM! He's in

sewer. *"How the hell did this happen again?!"* he exclaimed.
This time Joe figured out how to escape the sewer a bit faster,
and again swore to never let it happen again. Wednesday rolled
around and once again Joe found himself in the sewer. *"Ahhhhh!!*
OMG!! Not again!" Joe yelled with an increasing sense of
frustration. He quickly remembered how to get himself out and
continued on his way. On Thursday, as Joe walked down that
same street, something different happened. Right as he stepped
into the very same manhole, <u>he realized what was happening</u>. He
became aware of his mistake as he made the fatal error. He tried
to step back but it was too late, and into the sewer he went. **On**
Friday Joe was ready. He confidently strolled down the street,
and as he approached that manhole, he stopped himself one step
short. No sewer for Joe today. *He finally learned his lesson.*

Falling into the sewer is a metaphor for our automatic emotional
responses and decisions. These are not things we consciously *think*
about. Emotions often seem to have powers of their own, and only after
they arise (aka- falling into the sewer) do you get the opportunity to
address them. Like it or not we are emotional creatures. It is supremely
important to understand the power our emotions carry in daily decision

making processes, particularly in what we eat (or don't eat). Emotional intelligence will be one of your most powerful tools as you move forward with the *Eat Fat, Get Fit* program. But you may ask, *what does emotional intelligence mean?*

EMOTIONAL AWARENESS

The first step towards intelligence is awareness. We all carry within us years of emotional baggage. Some of it came from when we were kids, unbeknownst to us. I was a heavy soda drinker and developed a strong emotional connection to Coca-Cola. If I ever had a hard day, was stressed out, tired, angry, you name it, I reached for a Coke and it would instantly make me *feel* better. Take a moment to think about something that makes you feel better after a long day or a stressful situation. Pizza, beer, and cookies are common comfort foods for many.

Becoming aware of your emotional patterns and triggers is what will ultimately free you from them. Unfortunately, you may have to "fall in the sewer" a bunch of times before your emotional awareness really kicks in. Let's have a look at a common emotional trigger: STRESS. Everyone knows this trigger, but not many understand its power.

Imagine standing in line at the grocery store after a brutal day at the office. Your mind is racing, you feel physically tired, and all you want is to be on your couch relaxing. As you put the groceries on the conveyer belt, you catch a glimpse of the candy bars. *"One candy bar can't be that bad right?"* you say to yourself as you reach for the Snickers bar.

SPLASH! You just fell in the sewer.

Next, you are out to dinner with friends or family, someone tells you about the huge raise they just got. Your mind instantly thinks about all your bills and how it *feels* like there is never enough money. The bread basket comes around, and you grab two pieces.

"How the hell did I fall in the sewer again?" you'll say.

Two days later your spouse or significant other brings home one of those glorious pink boxes of donuts. The kids are beyond excited. *"I know I'm not supposed to...but I'll just have one"* you tell yourself. *"I've been good the past few days."* Suddenly, you are in the sewer again.

"HOW THE F$% DOES THIS KEEP HAPPENING???"* you scream at yourself. Splinter from the Ninja Turtles shakes his head as he walks by...

The following week that same box of donuts finds its way to your office kitchen, but something *feels* different. You've seen this before. You know what that pretty pink box means, and you know where it leads. You remember how you *felt* when Splinter walked by and gave you a disappointed look. Suddenly you realize, Splinter wasn't disappointed in you, it was **your** disappointment in **yourself** that you felt.

As a test of self control, you open the box, just to take a peek. It's like a scene from the movies when the pearly gates of Heaven open up. Beautiful bright lights come pouring out of the box as Angels sing majestically in the background. The donuts literally *feel* like Heaven. *"Not today"* you say, cracking a smile as you close the box. You *almost* fell into the sewer again but caught yourself just in the nick-of-time. <u>Your emotional awareness has expanded</u>. Splinter nods with approval from the sewer below as you reach for the healthy snack you brought from home.

Now this doesn't mean you won't end up in the sewer again. In fact it may take several more trips down the manhole before you finally grasp what is happening. The most important thing you can do after successfully stopping a plunge into the sewer is to **give yourself recognition**. Be **proud** of your accomplishment. Write it down. Tell someone about it! They may look at you funny but who cares!? This is truly a big moment in your life.

Emotional awareness is a tool 99% of other programs fail to give. Being emotional creatures, we must address this component of diet. This is what sets *Eat Fat, Get Fit apart from the rest*. Acknowledging your emotional patterns and triggers will ultimately lead to freedom from them. But acknowledgement can only come from awareness, so you will first need to become aware you are in the sewer before you can get yourself out.

KEY POINTS

- ➢ Emotions play an enormous role is our food choices
- ➢ Most emotional reactions and decisions are UNCONSCIOUS
  - ○ They occur without us actually thinking about them
- ➢ Becoming aware of our emotional patterns is the first step towards conquering them
- ➢ It make take weeks of trying before you notice them
- ➢ Be sure to PRAISE yourself when you uncover emotional triggers

➤ Do not beat yourself up when you are overcome by

them

   ○ This is totally normal and TO BE EXPECTED

   ○ Try laughing about it

15. Squash Social Pressure

We are social creatures. We like to talk to each other, to share our stories and experiences. We gather at sporting events, for dinner on a Friday, or church on Sunday. We talk about work, relationships, the game last night, and our families. We love to talk, and we do. Even if you don't, many people do. With this social dynamic often comes social pressures and opinions. For example; everyone loves to give their opinions. In many cases, it seems like an automatic "knee-jerk" response, as if the person showering you with their opinion can't stop even if they wanted. This can be particularly frustrating when someone feels the need give you their opinion about what *you are doing*, specifically when they tell you they think it's wrong or stupid.

As you follow the *Eat Fat, Get Fit* program, you will almost certainly encounter social situations that produce uncomfortable feelings. These interactions can make you feel uncomfortable with your choices and halt progress for those who aren't prepared. Let's walk through two typical scenarios people encounter while attempting to change their eating habits. Imagine being out to dinner with the guys and the waiter comes by to take your order:

Friend #1 - *"I'll have the patty-melt on sourdough with a Bud-Light."*

Friend #2 - *"I'm gonna get the blue cheese burger and a Coke."*

Friend #3 - *"The margarita pizza sounds amazing. I'll have that and a….Heineken."*

You - *"I'll have the bacon burger…and….uh…can you wrap it in lettuce instead of a bun?"*

The chattering stops and everyone looks your way…

You - *"And uh…a side salad. Water is fine to drink. Thanks!"*

Friend #2 - *"No bun on your burger!?!? The bun is the best part!!"*

Friend #1 - *"Please bring this guy a basket of bread when you come back with those Beers."*

Embarrassment levels can get high in situations like this. Many guys can relate, and for some, these moments can be the hardest obstacles to overcome. Women also run into complicated social settings. This is an example my wife ran into during her journey:

"I didn't want to eat the bread but I still did anyways! I was too nervous to order the lettuce wrap burger because I didn't want to have to explain myself to anyone if they asked me about it!"

113

Squashing social pressure involves accepting that other people have their own opinions. The only thing we can do about this is to be prepared for when they share them. To squash social pressure means to no longer be worried about what other people think of *your choices*. For many this can be difficult. In the early stages of my own weight-loss journey I caught myself being very concerned with what my friends and family thought of my choices! Only after several social interactions where I felt embarrassed and uncertain was I able to overcome this roadblock to success.

Other people may also tell you what you're doing is dangerous, unhealthy, or irresponsible. *"Did you know heart disease is the #1 killer in America? I don't think it's a good idea to be eating more fat. You have kids to worry about"* says Steven. Can you feel the **doubt** creeping in the back of your mind? I mean, Steven's brother is a doctor! He would know these things for sure! Right?!

What Steven doesn't understand is that you are already aware heart disease is the #1 killer in America. That is precisely why you are increasing fat intake and reducing simple carbohydrate consumption. Heart disease became the #1 killer of Americans at the same time we reduced dietary fat intake. They have occurred simultaneously; in tandem. Understanding this chain of events will catapult you over these types of social hurdles.

To sum it up, other people are going to have opinions about what you do. This is the way life works. How you <u>react</u> to their opinions is the only thing you have control over. You must learn to summon your inner confidence and be willing to confront these social situations if you are going to squash them. The next time you decide to skip dessert and someone says; *"Come on...live a little!"* you can kindly remind them you plan on living *more* than just a little.

KEY POINTS

- ➤ Social settings can be difficult in the beginning
- ➤ Being PREPARED for these or other scenarios will help you make the right choices and stick to your guns when the time comes
- ➤ Some people may call what you are doing *dangerous* or *irresponsible*
    - ○ The only thing you can do is allow them to have their opinions

- o Always remember why you are doing this in the first place
- ➢ Heart disease, cancer, and many other diseases have been on the rise at the same time our society cut fat and increased carbs
  - o They have happened simultaneously

16. Visualize Your Success

We always want the best tools for a job. The painter wants a high quality power-sprayer, the mechanic wants a hydraulic lift to easily get under the car, and the maid wants the best cleaning supplies. The right tools make any job easier. And guess what? **Losing weight is a job**. Just like painting a house, changing a car's oil, or cleaning the kitchen, it's a job that must be done. And, like the others, if it doesn't get done, problems may arise in the future. As you tackle the complicated job of weight-loss, you will find it much easier if you have the right tools for this job.

One of the newest tools for your "weight-loss tool belt" is **visualization**. Commonly thought of as hippy-nonsense, visualization has been validated by ultra successful individuals from every facet of life. Olympic gold medalist's and NBA all-stars incorporate visualization practices in order to perform and succeed under extreme pressure. Elite personal trainers have their clients visualizing their desired results alongside exercise routines in order to ensure a steady rate of progress.

HOW THIS WORKS

We all want to lose weight and get in great shape, but why is it so hard? Simply put, rules are hard to follow, hard to remember, and sometimes a funnel cake smells like heaven...literally. Our subconscious minds often get overwhelmed and forget about our desire to get in shape. We have so many thoughts running around our brains it becomes easy to lose sight of what's **really** important.

Visualizing your future fitness accomplishments sends a powerful message to your subconscious mind about what you think is truly important. Sending these repeated messages to your subconscious will help to make better decisions in the future. You may reach for a candy bar in the grocery store checkout and suddenly pull back because you *remember* that candy does not actually give you what you want. Your subconscious will remember what you consciously want; health, fitness, and happiness.

The following are three exercises to use in order to help ensure your success in following the *Eat Fat, Get Fit* program:

EXERCISE 1:

Make sure you are in a comfortable place with no distractions. Close your eyes and imagine your desired physical appearance. Picture your muscles, complexion, and weight. Really soak in this future version of yourself. Where are you? What are you wearing? Are you at the beach in a bikini or the gym in a tank top? The goal here is to make it as <u>descriptive as possible</u>. Once per day is an excellent starting point, but feel free to do it as often as you like. The more the better.

EXERCISE 2:

Again, make sure you are in a comfortable place with no distractions. Close your eyes and envision a scenario where you are offered a food or drink you wish to avoid. Put yourself at a dinner party, family gathering, a bar, restaurant, or any place you will be confronted with temptation. Visualize yourself declining bread as your appetizer. *How* do you decline? Do you smile and say no thank you? Reel in horror? Do you look nervous? Confident? Really play through this future moment and its different possibilities. Remember, while you may be saying "no" to bread, you are actually saying "yes" to your health. Do this daily as well.

EXERCISE 3:

With a pen a paper handy, imagine sitting down with your future self who has already achieved your health and fitness goals. Your future self might have a shredded 6-pack or the perfect bikini-bod, or maybe their diabetes or hypothyroidism as been cured.

Whatever it is you currently desire. **Ask your future self for the top three tips which helped him or her achieve their success. Write these tips down.** By doing this you have effectively given yourself advice from the future. Look at these tips daily as a reminder of the goals you wish to accomplish, and <u>follow the advice</u> from your future self.

After you can easily visualize these in detail, use your newly found imagination to come up with other similar visualization scenarios. Visualizing is not mandatory, and you can still achieve your desired results without it. It is simply a tool to help you finish your weight-loss job. My own weight-loss occurred *before* I learned of the power of visualization. However, had I known of its power to help, I would have surely used it, possibly saving an enormous amount of time and energy that was wasted fighting with myself.

For more information on visualization and mediation practices visit: www.journeyofselflove.com

KEY POINTS

> **Visualization is a TOOL for you to use for your weight-loss job.**

- o This tool has recently become more understood and scientifically accepted
- ➤ Visualizing helps communicate your <u>conscious goals</u> to your <u>unconscious mind</u>
  - o It is like prep work for future situations
- ➤ Learning to say no *BEFORE* the candy isle is extremely powerful
- ➤ DO THE EXERCISES
  - o This is not mandatory but will dramatically increase your chances of success

17. Overcoming Your Fat Failures

Success is determined by your ability to overcome failure. This cannot be stressed enough. The road to high-fat success is tricky and filled with unexpected bumps and turns. In a matter of minutes you can find yourself speeding backwards away from your goals and towards your starting line. What you must understand is that this is <u>part of the process</u>. You are destined to run into moments of "failure" that must be overcome. **<u>How many times you overcome these "failures" will ultimately determine your level of success</u>**.

You may not *intentionally* ignore the advice given in this book, but if you lack a clear path to follow, back-steps will occur. Creating your new path takes more than just reading this book; it takes <u>practicing</u> what the book says to do. No one is good at anything without practice. The professional baseball player, the Broadway opera singer, and the late night talk show host have all endured countless failures in their journey to the top. When you run into these roadblocks to success it is imperative you remember one thing: **YOU HAVE THE CHOICE TO KEEP PUSHING FORWARD.** Keep in mind; nothing worth having is easy. If it was, everyone would have it.

Your path to high-fat, low-carb success may be littered with empty candy wrappers and pizza crusts. You may cry yourself to sleep over a pint of ice cream or eat four chilidogs at the baseball game. These are the speed bumps of your journey; bumps in the road to success. The most important thing to remember is **YOU MUST NEVER GIVE UP**. Only when you give up have you failed.

During times of doubt, remind yourself of WHY you want to *Eat Fat, Get Fit*. After every cheat meal, every holiday splurge, and every collapse in willpower, you must get up, wipe the bread crumbs from your face, and continue down your path to fat success. You will notice over time your path will become less bumpy and littered with candy wrappers and soda cans. Progress can be slow at times, but remember permanent weight-loss is a marathon not a sprint. <u>Slow and steady often wins the race.</u>

The final secret to fat success is to understand you are simply trying to improve upon the person you were yesterday. This competition with yourself will ultimately lead you to any physical or mental goals you have. Remember to cut yourself some slack and commend your successes as you overcome your failures.

KEY POINTS

- ➤ Be flexible with your "failures"

    - ○ Failure is only real if you don't learn from the experience

- ➤ You will ignore/forget this information in the <u>beginning</u>

    - ○ **THIS IS PART OF THE PLAN**

    - ○ Accept this and keep moving forward

- ➤ <u>Nothing worth having is easy</u>

A Fat Farewell

Before we part ways I would like to acknowledge you for taking the time to read this book. It shows you desire growth and are willing to work to achieve it. It is the work you put in that will ultimately give you the success you desire. Even if the *Eat Fat, Get Fit* program is not for you, it is clear you will find something that is, <u>and you will succeed.</u> If you do decide on a different approach, let me leave you with this:

> ***"The problem is we are not eating food anymore...we are eating food-like products"*** -Dr. Alejandro Junger

Frequently eating things that are *food-like* will steal your health, energy, memory, and years if not decades of your life. Within Dr. Junger's statement is a foundational principle of *Eat Fat, Get Fit*. Wherever your health and fitness journey takes you next, **bring his statement with you**. Internalize it. With each meal comes an opportunity for growth; for change. It is my hope this book has given you the ability to see opportunity where you once thought there was none, and that you apply these principles to help you grow into your ideal self. Your best self.

Good luck!

Eat Fat, Get Fit Comprehensive Foods Guide

- ❖ Eat as much healthy fats and vegetables per day as desired
- ❖ Moderate protein intake to one/two servings per meal (depending on fitness level)
- ❖ Moderate Dairy to one/two serving per day
- ❖ Eat fruits at night
- ❖ Eat carbs/starches at night after fitness training
- ❖ Eat when hungry and until you are full
- ❖ Drink enough water that urine is semi clear/odorless
- ❖ Organic, locally sourced, in season foods are optimal

Healthy Fats

Eat Freely:

- Coconut Oil
- Coconut milk/cream
- MCT oil
- Olive Oil
- Grass-fed Butter
- Sardines, Oysters (canned in olive oil)
- Pasture raised eggs
- Grass-fed beef, bison, lamb
- Olives
- Avocados
- Macadamia Nut oil
- Avocado Oil
- Ghee
- Cod liver oil, triglyceride based fish oil

- Grass-fed dairy (cheese, sour cream, cream cheese – Preferably raw)
- Bacon (uncured, sugar free, yeast extract free, celery extract free)
- Unsweetened nut butters (almond, cashew, walnut etc)
- Dark Chocolate (low sugar)

AVOID:
- Canola oil
- Vegetable Oil
- Roasted nuts and seeds
- Peanut butter
- Regular commercial butter
- Regular commercial (non grass-fed dairy)
- Non organic/pasture raised-grass-fed meats
- Margarine
- Farm-raised fish
- Safflower/sunflower oil
- Flax oil
- Soy
- Milk Chocolate
- Trans fats
- Commercially Fried foods
- Commercial bacon
- Processed meats (regular hot dogs, lunch meats, salami)

Vegetables

Eat Freely:
- Kale (preferably not raw – lightly steamed or cooked)
- Spinach
- Swiss chard
- Arugula
- Brussels Sprouts
- Broccoli
- Asparagus

- Bok Choy
- Leeks
- Cabbage (raw and cooked)
- Cauliflower
- Collard Greens
- Dandelion Greens
- Wheat Grass
- Nori (seaweed)
- Celery
- Cucumber

Moderate:
- Sweet potatoes (eat with fat)
- Squash
- Zucchini
- Carrots
- Romaine lettuce
- Red/butter lettuce
- Iceberg lettuce
- Radish

AVOID:
- Canned Vegetables
- Frozen Vegetables

Proteins

Eat Freely:
- Pasture raised eggs (with yolk)
- Grass-fed/pasture raised red meat (lamb, beef, bison, Elk, Venison)
- Organic Pork
- Wild Caught fish
- Goat Whey Protein Powder
- Raw Cheese (pasture raised/Grass-fed)

- Raw Milk (pasture raised/Grass-fed)
- Nuts – macadamia, pistachio, brazil (in shell), walnut, pecan, cashew
- Seeds – Hemp, Pepitas (pumpkin seeds), chia seeds

Moderate:
- Yogurt (full fat, organic, pasture raised or grass-fed)
- Dried, smoked meats (no nitrates, no MSG, no yeast extract, No celery extract)
- Cottage Cheese
- Egg protein powder
- Whey protein powder supplements
- Commercial non pasture raised eggs

AVOID:
- Commercial/non organic/non grass-fed dairy
- Commercial/non organic/non grass-fed meat
- Processed Cheeses
- Processed meats
- Soy
- Protein powders with sweeteners
- Casein Protein
- Muscle Milk

Starches

Eat Semi-Freely:
- Sweet potatoes (eat with fat)
- Soaked Wild Rice (rinsed thoroughly)
- Soaked Sushi rice (rinsed thoroughly)
- Soaked Brown Rice (rinsed thoroughly)
- Sprouted quinoa, legumes(beans/lentils), millet

Moderate:
- Non Soaked rice

- Soaked quinoa, legumes, millet
- Gluten free oats (steel cut)
- Sprouted wheat
- Rice Pasta/noodle
- Quinoa Pasta/noodle

AVOID:
- Gluten containing carbohydrates
- Non sprouted wheat/whole grain products
- Processed oats (Quaker style)
- Breads
- Pastas
- Corn
- Soy

Fruit

Eat Freely:
- Blueberries
- Raspberries
- Blackberries
- Cherries
- Strawberries
- Lemon
- Lime
- Grapefruit
- Kiwi
- Apples

Moderate:
- Mangoes
- Nectarines
- Peach
- Papaya
- Pears

- Pineapple
- Plumb
- Watermelon
- Grapes
- Dates
- Figs
- Melon/Cantaloupe

AVOID:
- Canned fruit
- Fruit snacks
- Fruit juices
- Smoothies with added sugar
- Fruit juice
- Fruit in syrup
- Sugar added dried fruit

Spices/Seasonings/Sweeteners

Eat Freely:
- Cinnamon
- Organic Vanilla Extract
- Turmeric
- Cumin
- Cardamom
- Curry
- Cayenne
- Fennel
- Star anise
- Garlic
- Ginger
- Fenugreek
- Cloves
- Stevia
- Celtic Sea Salt

- Himalayan Salt
- Braggs Liquid Aminos
- Coconut Aminos
- Apple Cider Vinegar

Moderate:
- Raw Honey
- Coconut Nectar
- Regular table salt
- Pepper
- Garlic salt (if contains unknown ingredients)

AVOID:
- Sugar
- High Fructose Corn Syrup
- Regular Honey
- Agave Nectar
- Aspartame
- Soda
- MSG
- Salad dressing (unknown ingredients)

Drinks

Consume Freely:
- Purified water
- Mineral water (San Pellegrino/Perrier – lemon/lime/grapefruit flavors are ok)
- Lemon Water/Lime Water
- Water with added effervescent tablet (Nuun brand)
- Kombucha
- Raw Milk
- Coconut water (moderate)

Energy Drinks

Moderate:
- Organic Coffee
- Organic black/green/grey teas
- Yerba Matte
- 5 hour energy

Alcohol

Moderate:
- Clear tequila
- Potato vodka
- Gin (mixed with club soda/mineral water/lemon/lime)

AVOID:
- Mixed drinks
- Beer
- Red bull/monster/redline/amped/etc
- Any soda
- Smoothies
- Tap water

RESOURCES

Introduction

1. US Department of Agriculture. Web. <https://fnic.nal.usda.gov/how-many-calories-are-one-gram-fat-carbohydrate-or-protein>
2. Ingraham, Christopher. "The average American woman no weight as much as the average 1960s man" Washington Post. Web. June, 2016. <https://www.washingtonpost.com/news/wonk/wp/2015/06/12/look-at-how-much-weight-weve-gained-since-the-1960s/>

Chapter 1: A Very Fat History

1. Hyman M.D., Mark. Eat Fat, Get Thin: Why the Fat We Eat Is the Key to Sustained Weight Loss and Vibrant Health. Little, Brown and Company. Kindle Edition.
2. May AL, Kuklina EV, Yoon PW. Prevalence of cardiovascular disease risk factors among US adolescents, 1999– 2008. Pediatrics. 2012 Jun; 129(6): 1035– 41.

Chapter 2: Fear Behind The Fat

1. Think Organic Food is expensive? Huffington Post. <http://images.huffingtonpost.com/2015-10-05-1444073091-7683274-obese.gif> 2015 Oct. Web.
2. Am J Clin Nutr. 2010 Mar;91(3):535-46. doi: 10.3945/ajcn.2009.27725. Epub 2010 Jan 13. Meta-analysis of prospective cohort studies evaluating the association of saturated fat with cardiovascular disease. Siri-Tarino PW1, Sun Q, Hu FB, Krauss RM.
3. Barclay AW, Petocz P, McMillan-Price J, et al. Glycemic index, glycemic load, and chronic disease risk— a meta-analysis of observational studies. Am J Clin Nutr. 2008 Mar; 87(3): 627– 37. Review.
4. J Nutr. 2015 Feb;145(2):299-305. doi: 10.3945/jn.114.203505. Epub 2014 Dec 10. Dietary intake of saturated fat is not associated with risk of coronary events or mortality in patients with established coronary artery disease. Puaschitz, Strand, Norekvål 3, Dierkes, Dahl, Svingen, Assmus, Schartum-Hansen H6, Øyen Pedersen, Drevon, Nygård

Chapter 3: Satan's Sweet Tooth

1. Daily bingeing on sugar repeatedly releases dopamine in the accumbens shell. Rada P1, Avena NM, Hoebel BG. Neuroscience. 2005;134(3):737-44.

2. Emotions & Blood-Sugar Levels: How Diabetes Can Affect Your Mood. Joslin Diabetes Center <http://blog.joslin.org/2014/07/emotions-blood-sugar-levels-how-diabetes-can-affect-your-mood-2/>

3. NIH study shows how insulin stimulates fat cells to take in glucose. NIH News Releases. Sept 7, 2010. < https://www.nih.gov/news-events/news-releases/nih-study-shows-how-insulin-stimulates-fat-cells-take-glucose>

Chapter 4: Good Fat Bad Fat?

1. Boyd, Tim. "FAQ-Dairy." *The Weston A. Price* Foundation. 6 Mar 2009. Web. 6 Feb 2015. <http://www.westonaprice.org/health-topics/faq-dairy/>

2. A. J. McAfee, E. M. McSorley, G. J. Cuskelly, A. M. Fearon, B. W. Moss, J. A. M. Beattie, J. M. W. Wallace, M. P. Bonham and J. J. Strain (2011). Red meat from animals offered a grass diet increases plasma and platelet n-3 PUFA in healthy consumers. British Journal of Nutrition, 105, pp 80-89. doi:10.1017/S0007114510003090.

3. Factory Farming and Human Health. <http://www.farmsanctuary.org/learn/factory-farming/factory-farming-and-human-health/>

4. 4. Dhiman, T. R., G. R. Anand, *et al.* (1999). "Conjugated linoleic acid content of milk from cows fed different diets." J Dairy Sci 82(10): 2146-56.

5. Wellness Mama. *The Importance of Soaking Nuts & Seeds*. Web. <http://wellnessmama.com/59139/soaking-nuts-seeds/>

6. Dr. Oz: The Secrets the Nut Industry Doesn't Want You to Know. 7/9/2012. Web <http://www.doctoroz.com/blog/daniel-heller-nd/secrets-nut-industry-doesnt-want-you-know>

7. Nazaryan, Claudette. Benefits of Pure Cold-Pressed Coconut Oil. SF Gate < http://healthyeating.sfgate.com/benefits-pure-coldpressed-coconut-oil-7169.html>

8. https://en.wikipedia.org/wiki/Olive_oil_extraction

9. Michel de Lorgeril and Patricia Salen . *New insights into the health effects of dietary saturated and omega-6 and omega-3 polyunsaturated fatty acids.* BMC Medicine201210:50 DOI: 10.1186/1741-7015-10-50 ©de Lorgeril and Salen; licensee BioMed Central Ltd. 2012 Received: 17 February 2012Accepted: 21 May 2012Published: 21 May 2012

10. Conjugated Linoleic Acid Decreases MCF-7 Human Breast Cancer Cell Growth and Insulin-Like Growth Factor-1 Receptor Levels. Danielle L. Amarù, Catherine J. Field. Lipids. May 2009, Volume 44, Issue 5, pp 449-458

11. Conjugated Linoleic Acid (CLA) Up-regulates the Estrogenregulated Cancer Suppressor Gene, Protein Tyrosine Phosphatase Á (PTPÁ), in Human Breast Cells LI-SHU WANG1, YI-WEN HUANG1, YASURO SUGIMOTO1,2, SULING LIU3, HSIANG-LIN CHANG1, WEIPING YE1, SHERRY SHU1 and YOUNG C. LIN1,2. International Journal of Cancer Research and Treatment.

12. The FASEB Journal express article 10.1096/fj.00-0359fje. Published online October 6, 2000. Anti-inflammatory effects of sodium butyrate on human monocytes: potent inhibition of IL-12 and up-regulation of IL-10 production Marcus D. Säemann, Georg A. Böhmig, Christoph H. Österreicher, Helmut Burtscher,Ornella Parolini, Christos Diakos, Johannes Stöckl, Walter H. Hörl, and Gerhard J.Zlabinger

13. Scand J Gastroenterol. 2002 Apr;37(4):458-66. Butyrate inhibits NF-kappaB activation in lamina propria macrophages of patients with ulcerative colitis. Lührs H1, Gerke T, Müller JG, Melcher R, Schauber J, Boxberge F, Scheppach W, Menzel T. PMID: 11989838

14. Diabetes. 2009 Jul; 58(7): 1509–1517. Published online 2009 Apr 14. doi: 10.2337/db08-1637 PMCID: PMC2699871 Butyrate Improves Insulin Sensitivity and Increases Energy Expenditure in Mice Zhanguo Gao,1 Jun Yin,1 Jin Zhang,1 Robert E. Ward,2 Roy J. Martin,1 Michael Lefevre,2 William T. Cefalu,1 and Jianping Ye1

Chapter 5: Meat, Dairy, and Eggs

1. Environmental Medicine, Part 1: The Human Burden of Environmental Toxins and Their Common Health Effects by Walter J. Crinnion, ND, Alternative Medicine Review, Volume 5 Number 1, 2000, page52

2. Dhiman, T. R., G. R. Anand, *et al.* (1999). "Conjugated linoleic acid content of milk from cows fed different diets." J Dairy Sci 82(10): 2146-56.

3. A. J. McAfee, E. M. McSorley, G. J. Cuskelly, A. M. Fearon, B. W. Moss, J. A. M. Beattie, J. M. W. Wallace, M. P. Bonham and J. J. Strain (2011). Red meat from animals offered a grass diet increases plasma and platelet n-3 PUFA in healthy consumers. British Journal of Nutrition, 105, pp 80-89. doi:10.1017/S0007114510003090.

4. Barrionuevo, Alexei. "Salmon Virus Indicts Chile's Fishing Methods." *The New Your Times*. 27 March 2008. Web. 22 Feb 2015. <http://www.nytimes.com/2008/03/27/world/americas/27salmon.html?adxnnl=1&adxnnlx=1423663240-kMSlt7tO0y2buv/RvIveQg&_r=0>.

5. Farmed and Dangerous. FAQ. Web http://www.farmedanddangerous.org/salmon-farming-problems/frequently-asked-questions/

6. Free aromatic amino acids in egg yolk show antioxidant properties. Chamila Nimalaratne, Daise Lopes-Lutz, Andreas Schieber, Jianping Wu, Department of Agricultural, Food and Nutritional Science (AFNS), 4-10 Ag/For Centre, University of Alberta, Edmonton, Alberta, Canada T6G 2P5. doi:10.1016/j.foodchem.2011.04.058

7. Lundell, Dwight; Nordstrom, Todd. The Cure for Heart Disease: Truth Will Save a Nation (Kindle Location 203). Kindle Edition.

8. Long, Cheryl. Mother Earth News. *Meet Real Free-Range Eggs.* Nov. 2007. <http://www.motherearthnews.com/real-food/free-range-eggs-zmaz07onzgoe.aspx#axzz2Og4gJemy>

Chapter 6: The Calorie Myth

1. Merriam-Webster. Calorie. <http://www.merriam-webster.com/dictionary/calorie>

2. Wikipedia. Calorimeter. <https://en.wikipedia.org/wiki/Calorimeter>

3. WebMD. Your Digestive System. <http://www.webmd.com/heartburn-gerd/your-digestive-system>

Chapter 7: Sugar vs. Fat: The Energy Showdown

1. https://en.wikipedia.org/wiki/Hypoglycemia

2. https://en.wikipedia.org/wiki/Ketosis

Chapter 8: Becoming Fat Adapted

1. Stein, E. *Ketogenic Catastrophe: Avoid The Ketogenic Diet Mistakes.* Disruptive Publishing 2015. Print (P.14-17)

Chapter 9: Turbocharged Weight Loss

1. NIH study shows how insulin stimulates fat cells to take in glucose. NIH News Releases. Sept 7, 2010. < https://www.nih.gov/news-events/news-releases/nih-study-shows-how-insulin-stimulates-fat-cells-take-glucose>
2. Gardner CD, Kiazand A, Alhassan S, et al. Comparison of the Atkins, Zone, Ornish, and LEARN diets for change in weight and related risk factors among overweight premenopausal women: the A TO Z Weight Loss Study: a randomized trial. JAMA. 2007 Mar 7;297(9): 969– 77.

Chapter 10: A New World of Physical Performance

1. Lundell, Dwight; Nordstrom, Todd. The Cure for Heart Disease: Truth Will Save a Nation (Kindle Location 203). Kindle Edition.
2. Caldwell, Emily. Ohio State University News Room. *Endurance athletes who 'go against the grain' become incredible fat-burners*. Web. Nov 2015. <https://news.osu.edu/news/2015/11/16/against-grain/>
3. Barañano KW, Hartman AL. The Ketogenic Diet: Uses in Epilepsy and Other Neurologic Illnesses. Current treatment options in neurology. 2008;10(6):410-419.
4. Department of Molecular Pharmacology and Physiology, Morsani College of Medicine. *Ketone supplementation decreases tumor cell viability and prolongs survival of mice with metastatic cancer.* A.M. Poff , C. Ari, P. Arnold, T.N. Seyfried and D.P. D'Agostino. Hyperbaric Biomedical Research Laboratory, University of South Florida, Tampa, FL Savind, Inc., Seymour, IL Department of Biology, Boston College, Chestnut Hill, MA
5. Dr. Mercola, Joseph. *Why Exercise and Endorphins Make You Happy.* <http://fitness.mercola.com/sites/fitness/archive/2016/01/29/exercise-endorphins-happiness.aspx> Web.

Chapter 11: Get Smart and Sexy - How Fat Improves Cognition

1. Berg JM, Tymoczko JL, Stryer L. Biochemistry. 5th edition. New York: W H Freeman; 2002. Section 30.2, Each Organ Has a Unique Metabolic Profile. Available from: http://www.ncbi.nlm.nih.gov/books/NBK22436/
2. LaManna JC, Salem N, Puchowicz M, et al. KETONES SUPPRESS BRAIN GLUCOSE CONSUMPTION. *Advances in experimental medicine and biology.* 2009;645:301-306. doi:10.1007/978-0-387-85998-9_45.

3. Roberts RO, Roberts LA, Geda YE, et al. Relative intake of macronutrients impacts risk of mild cognitive impairment or dementia. J Alzheimers Dis. 2012;32(2): 329– 39.
4. Barberger-Gateau P, Raffaitin C, Letenneur L, et al. Dietary patterns and risk of dementia: the three-city cohort study. Neurology. 2007 Nov 13;69(20): 1921– 30.
5. Valls-Pedret C, Sala-Vila A, Serra-Mir M, et al. Mediterranean diet and age-related cognitive decline: a randomized clinical trial. JAMA Intern Med. 2015 May 11.

www.ingramcontent.com/pod-product-compliance
Lightning Source LLC
Chambersburg PA
CBHW072050280526
45788CB00006B/2254